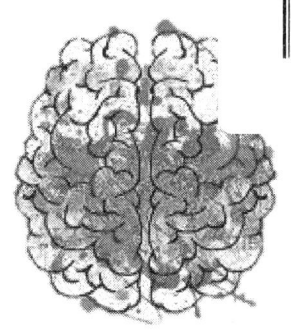

BEYOND DEMENTIA

"Understanding, Coping, and Thriving in the Face of Memory Loss"

MIKE STEVES

Edited by: Wilcox Samuel and Mark Russo

Design Layout: Joy Margaret

Copyright © [2024]. All rights reserved.

No part of this publication may be reproduced, distributed, or transmitted in any form or by any means, including photocopying, recording, or other electronic or mechanical methods, without the prior written permission of the publisher, except in the case of brief quotations embodied in critical reviews and certain other noncommercial uses permitted by copyright law.

TABLE OF CONTENTS

INTRODUCTION TO DEMENTIA 6
Overview and Definitions 9
Types of Dementia 13
Prevalence and Impact 17

THE BRAIN AND DEMENTIA 21
Anatomy of the Brain 22
How Dementia Affects the Brain 25
Neurological Basis of Dementia 30

TYPES OF DEMENTIA 35
Alzheimer's Disease 36
Vascular Dementia 41
Lewy Body Dementia 46
Frontotemporal Dementia 49
Other Forms of Dementia 55

RISK FACTORS AND CAUSES 60
Lifestyle and Environmental Factors 61
Comorbid Conditions 66

DIAGNOSIS AND EARLY DETECTION OF DEMENTIA 73

Symptoms and Early Signs 74
Diagnostic Procedures 79
Importance of Early Diagnosis 82

CARING FOR SOMEONE WITH DEMENTIA 86
Roles and Responsibilities of Caregivers 87
Daily Care Routines 91
Managing Stress and Caregiver Burnout 96

COMMUNICATION STRATEGIES 100
Effective Communication Techniques 101
Understanding Behavioral Changes 105
Maintaining Relationships 109

THERAPIES AND TREATMENTS 113
Pharmacological Treatments 114
Non-Pharmacological Approaches 117

PREVENTIVE STRATEGIES 123
Lifestyle Modifications 124
Public Health Initiatives 127
Education and Awareness Campaigns 131

CONCLUSION 135

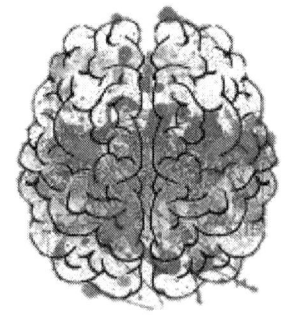

INTRODUCTION

A Journey into the Unknown

John Matthews was a man who epitomized strength, intellect, and kindness. A retired engineer, he spent his days tinkering with old clocks, a hobby that required precision and a keen eye for detail. His life was filled with love, surrounded by his wife of fifty years, their three children, and five grandchildren. To his family, John was a pillar of wisdom and a source of endless stories. He was the kind of grandfather who never missed a soccer game, who built elaborate treehouses, and who could fix anything that was broken.

One autumn afternoon, as the leaves turned shades of amber and gold, John found himself in his workshop, struggling to recall the intricate steps needed to repair a clock he had fixed countless times before. At first, he dismissed it as a fleeting lapse, the kind that happens to everyone now and then. However, the moments of forgetfulness became more frequent and more troubling. His once sharp mind seemed to be clouding over with a fog that he couldn't shake.

John's family began to notice subtle changes too. He repeated stories within minutes of telling them, misplaced everyday items, and often seemed confused in familiar settings. The man who had always been so sure of himself was becoming increasingly uncertain. Concerned, his wife, Margaret, convinced him to see a doctor. After a series of tests and evaluations, the diagnosis came: John had early-stage Alzheimer's disease, a form of dementia.

Understanding Dementia

Dementia is not a single disease but a collective term used to describe various symptoms of cognitive decline, such as memory loss, confusion, and impaired judgment. It encompasses several specific conditions, the most common being Alzheimer's disease, which accounts for 60-80% of cases. Other forms include vascular dementia, Lewy body dementia, and frontotemporal dementia. While each type affects the brain differently, they all share the devastating impact on an individual's ability to perform everyday activities.

The Prevalence and Impact

The reach of dementia is extensive and growing. Currently, over 50 million people worldwide are living with dementia, a number projected to triple by 2050 due to aging populations. It does not discriminate, affecting people across all walks of life, though age is the strongest risk factor. The condition brings not only emotional and physical strain on those diagnosed but also on their families and caregivers, who often bear the brunt of the caregiving responsibilities.

The Human Brain and Dementia

To comprehend dementia, it's essential to understand the brain's complexity. The brain, a marvel of nature, controls our thoughts, memories, emotions, and movements. In dementia, damage to brain cells interferes with their ability to communicate, affecting functions managed by different regions of the brain. Alzheimer's disease, for example, primarily affects the hippocampus, the area responsible for memory formation, explaining why memory loss is a hallmark symptom.

Risk Factors and Causes

Dementia arises from a combination of genetic, environmental, and lifestyle factors. While age and genetics are significant contributors, factors like smoking, diet, physical inactivity, and head injuries also play crucial roles. Comorbid conditions such as diabetes, hypertension, and cardiovascular diseases further increase the risk. Understanding these factors is vital in both prevention and management.

Diagnosis and Early Detection

Early detection of dementia can make a substantial difference in the management and progression of the disease. The diagnostic process typically involves a comprehensive evaluation, including medical history, physical examination, neurological tests, and brain imaging. Recognizing the early signs, such as memory lapses, difficulty with familiar tasks, and changes in mood or behavior, is critical for seeking timely medical advice.

Moving Forward

John Matthews' story is one among millions, a poignant reminder of the profound impact dementia can have on individuals and their loved ones. As we delve deeper into understanding this condition, the goal is not only to shed light on its complexities but also to foster empathy, awareness, and support for those affected. Through education, research, and compassionate care, we can hope to improve the quality of life for those living with dementia and their families, paving the way for a future where the shadow of dementia is significantly diminished.

Overview and Definitions

Dementia is a broad term for a range of conditions characterized by impairment in memory, thinking, behavior, and the ability to perform everyday activities. It is not a specific illness but rather a syndrome with multiple causes. This chapter provides an overview of dementia and its various definitions to help readers understand the scope and complexity of the condition.

Dementia involves a decline in cognitive function severe enough to interfere with daily life. It is caused by damage to brain cells, which impedes their ability to communicate effectively. This disruption in cellular communication leads to changes in behavior, emotions, and the overall functioning of an individual.

Several distinct types of dementia exist, each with unique features and progression patterns. The most prevalent form is Alzheimer's disease, responsible for the majority of cases. Vascular dementia, often resulting from strokes, involves issues with blood supply to the brain. Lewy body dementia is marked by abnormal protein deposits in nerve cells, while frontotemporal dementia affects the brain's frontal and temporal lobes, impacting personality and language.

Dementia symptoms vary but generally include memory loss, confusion, disorientation, and difficulty with communication and reasoning. As the condition advances, individuals may experience profound changes in personality and behavior, ultimately losing the ability to perform routine tasks independently.

It is crucial to differentiate between normal aging-related cognitive decline and dementia. While occasional forgetfulness and slower processing are common in older adults, dementia involves significant and progressive cognitive impairment that disrupts daily living. Recognizing these differences is essential for early diagnosis and intervention.

Dementia affects millions worldwide, with prevalence increasing with age. Although it primarily impacts older adults, younger individuals can also develop certain types. The condition poses a significant public health challenge, with rising numbers anticipated due to aging populations globally.

Several factors contribute to the likelihood of developing dementia, including age, genetics, and family history. Lifestyle choices such as diet, exercise, and cognitive engagement play a role in brain health. Conditions like hypertension, diabetes, and cardiovascular disease also increase risk. Identifying and managing these factors can help mitigate the risk.

Diagnosis involves a thorough assessment, including medical history, cognitive tests, neurological exams, and imaging studies. Early detection is vital for effective management and planning. Healthcare professionals use specific criteria and tools to evaluate cognitive function and determine the presence and type of dementia.

Currently, no cure exists for dementia, but treatments are available to manage symptoms and improve quality of life. Medications can alleviate some cognitive and behavioral symptoms, while non-pharmacological approaches, such as cognitive therapies, exercise, and social engagement, provide additional support. Comprehensive care involves addressing medical, psychological, and social needs.

Raising awareness about dementia is critical for early detection, reducing stigma, and providing better support for individuals and their families. Understanding the condition fosters empathy and encourages communities to develop dementia-friendly environments.

Dementia encompasses a range of conditions that profoundly impact individuals and society. By understanding its various types, symptoms, and risk factors, we can better support those affected and work towards improved treatments and care strategies. This chapter lays the foundation for a deeper exploration of dementia, guiding readers through its complexities and challenges.

Types of Dementia

Dementia encompasses a range of conditions characterized by cognitive decline and memory impairment. Each type has unique features, causes, and progression patterns. This chapter delves into the most common types, providing an in-depth understanding of their distinct characteristics.

Alzheimer's Disease

Overview: Alzheimer's disease is the most prevalent form of dementia, accounting for 60-80% of cases. It is marked by the gradual deterioration of brain cells, leading to memory loss, confusion, and difficulty with thinking and behavior.

Symptoms: Early symptoms include short-term memory loss, forgetting recent events or conversations, and difficulty finding words. As the disease progresses, individuals may experience severe memory loss, impaired reasoning, disorientation, mood swings, and changes in personality.

Causes: The exact cause is not fully understood, but it involves the accumulation of amyloid plaques and tau tangles in the brain. Genetic factors, such as mutations in specific genes (e.g., APOE4), and lifestyle factors also contribute.

Progression: Alzheimer's disease progresses slowly, with symptoms worsening over several years. It typically advances through stages, from mild cognitive impairment to moderate and severe dementia, ultimately leading to total dependence on caregivers.

Vascular Dementia

Overview: Vascular dementia results from impaired blood flow to the brain, often due to strokes or small vessel disease. It is the second most common type of dementia.

Symptoms: Symptoms vary depending on the brain region affected but often include confusion, difficulty with concentration, impaired judgment, and trouble with motor skills. Sudden onset or stepwise deterioration following strokes is common.

Causes: Risk factors include hypertension, diabetes, smoking, high cholesterol, and cardiovascular disease. These conditions damage blood vessels, leading to reduced blood flow and brain cell death.

Progression: The progression of vascular dementia can be stepwise, with periods of stability followed by sudden declines, especially after a stroke or other vascular events.

Lewy Body Dementia

Overview: Lewy body dementia (LBD) is characterized by abnormal deposits of a protein called alpha-synuclein in the brain. It includes two related conditions: dementia with Lewy bodies and Parkinson's disease dementia.

Symptoms: Key symptoms include fluctuating cognition, visual hallucinations, REM sleep behavior disorder, and parkinsonian motor symptoms (tremors, stiffness, slow movement). Individuals may also experience autonomic nervous system dysfunction, causing issues like blood pressure fluctuations and bowel problems.

Causes: The exact cause is unknown, but it is linked to the buildup of Lewy bodies. Genetic and environmental factors may play a role.

Progression: LBD progresses gradually, with cognitive and motor symptoms worsening over time. Fluctuations in alertness and severity of symptoms can occur daily.

Frontotemporal Dementia

Overview: Frontotemporal dementia (FTD) involves the degeneration of the frontal and temporal lobes of the brain, affecting personality, behavior, and language.

Symptoms: Early symptoms often include changes in personality and behavior, such as apathy, inappropriate social behavior, and loss of empathy. Language difficulties, including speaking and understanding speech, are also common.

Causes: FTD has a strong genetic component, with several genes (e.g., MAPT, GRN) linked to the disease. It can also occur sporadically without a known family history.

Progression: FTD typically progresses faster than Alzheimer's disease, with significant changes in personality and behavior appearing early. As the disease advances, individuals may lose the ability to speak and move.

Mixed Dementia

Overview: Mixed dementia involves a combination of two or more types of dementia, most commonly Alzheimer's disease and vascular dementia.

Symptoms: Symptoms reflect the types of dementia involved. For example, a person with mixed Alzheimer's and vascular dementia may exhibit memory loss and confusion alongside impaired judgment and motor skills.

Causes: The causes are a combination of factors from the involved types of dementia. For instance, amyloid plaques and tau tangles of Alzheimer's disease may coexist with vascular damage due to strokes or other vascular issues.

Progression: The progression of mixed dementia can vary but often includes elements of the diseases involved, leading to a complex and sometimes more rapid decline.

Other Forms of Dementia

Parkinson's Disease Dementia: This type of dementia develops in the later stages of Parkinson's disease, characterized by symptoms similar to Lewy body dementia, including motor symptoms, memory loss, and visual hallucinations.

Huntington's Disease: A genetic disorder causing the progressive breakdown of nerve cells in the brain, leading to dementia, movement disorders, and psychiatric symptoms.

Creutzfeldt-Jakob Disease: A rare, rapidly progressive disease caused by prion proteins, leading to dementia, motor dysfunction, and severe neurological decline.

Wernicke-Korsakoff Syndrome: Often linked to chronic alcoholism, this condition is caused by a deficiency in thiamine (vitamin B1), resulting in severe memory problems and neurological symptoms.

This comprehensive overview of the various types of dementia highlights the diversity of symptoms, causes, and progression patterns. Understanding these differences is crucial for accurate diagnosis, effective management, and providing appropriate care for individuals affected by dementia.

Prevalence and Impact

Dementia is a widespread and growing issue, affecting millions of individuals worldwide. As of recent estimates, over 50 million people live with dementia globally, a number that is expected to triple by 2050 due to increasing life expectancies and aging populations. This condition does not recognize borders, impacting every country and culture, although the prevalence rates can vary depending on demographic and socioeconomic factors.

While dementia affects people worldwide, its prevalence differs across regions. Higher-income countries typically report higher rates, partly due to better diagnostic capabilities and aging populations. However, low- and middle-income countries are experiencing rapid increases in cases, and by 2050, it is estimated that 68% of the global dementia population will be in these regions. This trend underscores the urgent need for global public health initiatives and resources to address the rising tide of dementia.

For those diagnosed with dementia, the impact is profound and multifaceted. Cognitive decline interferes with daily activities, leading to a loss of independence. Simple tasks like dressing, cooking, or managing finances become challenging, and in advanced stages, basic self-care abilities can be lost. Memory loss, confusion, and disorientation are common, often accompanied by changes in mood and behavior, such as increased anxiety, depression, and aggression. These changes can significantly diminish the quality of life, not only for those with the condition but also for their families and caregivers.

The emotional toll of dementia extends beyond cognitive symptoms. Individuals may experience a range of psychological effects, including frustration, fear, and sadness, as they grapple with the progressive loss of their abilities and sense of self. Relationships with family and friends can also be strained, as loved ones adjust to the changing dynamics and the person's shifting needs and behaviors.

Dementia also has a substantial social impact. Stigma and misunderstanding about the condition can lead to social isolation for those affected and their families. Communities may lack awareness and resources to support individuals with dementia, leading to a lack of appropriate care options and support networks. Social withdrawal is common as both patients and their caregivers might avoid public situations to manage symptoms privately.

The economic impact of dementia is staggering. Globally, the annual cost of dementia is estimated at over $1 trillion, a figure projected to rise dramatically. These costs include direct medical expenses, such as diagnosis, treatment, and long-term care, as well as indirect costs like lost productivity and informal care provided by family members. Many families face significant financial strain, as caregiving responsibilities often require them to reduce work hours or leave employment altogether.

Healthcare systems worldwide are grappling with the increasing demand for dementia care. This includes a need for more specialized healthcare professionals, improved diagnostic tools, and better long-term care facilities. Caregiving, typically provided by family members, is both physically and emotionally demanding. Caregivers often experience high levels of stress, burnout, and health problems due to the extensive demands of providing continuous care.

Addressing dementia poses numerous public health challenges. These include the need for early diagnosis and intervention, which can improve outcomes and quality of life for those affected. Public health initiatives must focus on awareness campaigns to reduce stigma and promote understanding. Additionally, research into prevention, treatment, and ultimately a cure is critical. Developing effective public policies and allocating resources to support dementia care and research are essential steps in managing the growing impact of this condition.

As life expectancy increases, the number of people living with dementia will continue to rise. Projections indicate that by 2050, the global dementia population will exceed 150 million. This anticipated growth highlights the urgent need for comprehensive strategies to address the medical, social, and economic challenges posed by dementia. Investment in research, support for caregivers, and the development of dementia-friendly communities will be crucial in mitigating the future impact.

The prevalence and impact of dementia are vast, affecting millions of individuals and their families worldwide. Understanding the scope of this condition is crucial for developing effective strategies to address its challenges, support those affected, and ultimately work towards reducing its global burden.

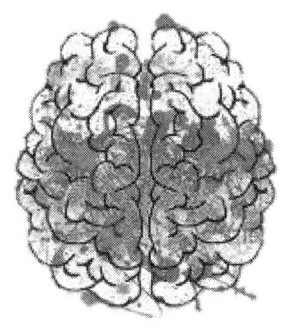

CHAPTER 1:

THE BRAIN AND DEMENTIA

Anatomy of the Brain

Understanding the anatomy of the brain is essential to grasp how dementia affects its function. The brain is a highly complex organ, responsible for controlling thoughts, emotions, movements, and numerous bodily functions. This chapter explores the key structures of the brain and their roles, highlighting how dementia disrupts these functions.

Overview of Brain Structure

The brain is divided into several regions, each with distinct functions. These regions include the cerebrum, cerebellum, and brainstem. The cerebrum is further divided into two hemispheres and four primary lobes: frontal, parietal, temporal, and occipital. Each part of the brain works in coordination with others to perform various tasks, from simple movements to complex cognitive processes.

The Cerebrum

Frontal Lobes: Located at the front of the brain, the frontal lobes are responsible for higher cognitive functions such as reasoning, planning, problem-solving, and controlling behavior and emotions. They also manage motor function and speech production through the primary motor cortex and Broca's area, respectively.

Parietal Lobes: Situated behind the frontal lobes, the parietal lobes process sensory information such as touch, temperature, and pain. They are crucial for spatial orientation and body awareness. The somatosensory cortex, located in the parietal lobes, helps integrate sensory input from different parts of the body.

Temporal Lobes: Found on the sides of the brain, near the temples, the temporal lobes are key for processing auditory information and are involved in memory formation. The hippocampus, located within the temporal lobes, plays a critical role in forming and retrieving memories. The temporal lobes also house Wernicke's area, essential for language comprehension.

Occipital Lobes: Located at the back of the brain, the occipital lobes are primarily responsible for visual processing. The primary visual cortex within these lobes interprets visual information received from the eyes.

The Cerebellum

The cerebellum, located under the cerebrum at the back of the brain, coordinates voluntary movements, balance, and posture. It ensures smooth and precise execution of motor activities by processing information from the sensory systems, spinal cord, and other parts of the brain.

The Brainstem

The brainstem, situated at the base of the brain, connects the brain to the spinal cord. It controls vital life functions such as breathing, heart rate, and blood pressure. The brainstem comprises three main parts: the midbrain, pons, and medulla oblongata. Each part plays a role in transmitting signals between the brain and the rest of the body.

Limbic System

The limbic system, a set of structures deep within the brain, regulates emotions, memory, and arousal. Key components of the limbic system include the hippocampus, amygdala, and hypothalamus.

Hippocampus: Essential for forming new memories and spatial navigation, the hippocampus is one of the first regions affected in Alzheimer's disease, leading to early memory loss.

Amygdala: Involved in processing emotions such as fear and pleasure, the amygdala also plays a role in memory consolidation, especially emotional memories.

Hypothalamus: The hypothalamus regulates autonomic functions such as hunger, thirst, body temperature, and circadian rhythms. It also controls the release of hormones from the pituitary gland.

Neurotransmitters and Brain Function

Neurons, the brain's nerve cells, communicate through chemical messengers called neurotransmitters. Several neurotransmitters are critical for normal brain function and are often disrupted in dementia.

Acetylcholine: Crucial for learning and memory, acetylcholine levels are significantly reduced in Alzheimer's disease, contributing to cognitive decline.

Dopamine: Involved in movement, motivation, and reward, dopamine dysregulation is a hallmark of Parkinson's disease and Lewy body dementia.

Serotonin: Regulates mood, sleep, and appetite. Changes in serotonin levels can affect behavior and mood in dementia patients.

Glutamate: The primary excitatory neurotransmitter, glutamate is essential for synaptic plasticity and cognitive functions. Excessive glutamate activity can lead to neuronal damage, observed in conditions like Alzheimer's disease.

How Dementia Affects the Brain

Dementia profoundly impacts the brain's structure and function, leading to the cognitive and behavioral symptoms associated with the condition. Each type of dementia has distinct pathological features, but they all involve the progressive degeneration of brain cells. This chapter delves into how dementia affects the brain at the cellular and systemic levels.

Cellular Changes in Dementia

Neuronal Death: The most fundamental change in dementia is the death of neurons, the brain's nerve cells. Neurons communicate through electrical and chemical signals, forming the basis of cognitive and motor functions. When these cells die, the brain's ability to process information deteriorates, leading to cognitive decline.

Synaptic Dysfunction: Synapses are the connections between neurons, allowing them to communicate. In dementia, synapses are often damaged or lost, disrupting neural networks and impairing cognitive functions such as memory, attention, and problem-solving.

Inflammation: Chronic inflammation is a common feature in many types of dementia. Microglia, the brain's immune cells, become overactive and release inflammatory cytokines, which can damage neurons and exacerbate neurodegeneration.

Alzheimer's Disease

Amyloid Plaques: One of the hallmarks of Alzheimer's disease is the accumulation of amyloid-beta protein outside neurons, forming sticky plaques. These plaques disrupt cell-to-cell communication and activate immune responses that lead to inflammation and neuronal death.

Tau Tangles: Inside neurons, tau proteins become abnormally phosphorylated and form twisted tangles. These tangles disrupt the transport of nutrients and other essential molecules within the cell, leading to cell death.

Brain Shrinkage: As neurons die and synapses are lost, the brain shrinks, particularly in the hippocampus and cortex. This atrophy correlates with the severity of cognitive decline and is visible in brain imaging studies.

Vascular Dementia

Reduced Blood Flow: Vascular dementia results from impaired blood flow to the brain, often due to strokes or small vessel disease. When brain cells do not receive enough oxygen and nutrients, they die, leading to cognitive deficits.

White Matter Lesions: Damage to the brain's white matter, which contains nerve fibers that connect different brain regions, is common in vascular dementia. This damage disrupts communication between brain regions, affecting cognitive and motor functions.

Lacunar Infarcts: Small strokes, known as lacunar infarcts, can occur in deep brain structures, causing localized damage and contributing to cognitive decline.

Lewy Body Dementia

Lewy Bodies: Lewy body dementia is characterized by the presence of Lewy bodies, abnormal aggregates of alpha-synuclein protein inside neurons. These inclusions disrupt normal cell function and lead to cell death.

Fluctuating Cognition: Lewy body dementia often causes rapid fluctuations in cognitive function, attention, and alertness. This variability is linked to the widespread distribution of Lewy bodies in different brain regions.

Visual Hallucinations: Lewy bodies in the visual processing areas of the brain can cause vivid visual hallucinations, a common symptom of this type of dementia.

Frontotemporal Dementia

Lobe-Specific Degeneration: Frontotemporal dementia involves the degeneration of the frontal and temporal lobes. This degeneration leads to significant changes in personality, behavior, and language, depending on which regions are affected.

Behavioral Changes: Damage to the frontal lobes, responsible for executive functions and social behavior, results in disinhibition, apathy, and impulsivity.

Language Impairments: When the temporal lobes are affected, individuals may experience primary progressive aphasia, characterized by difficulty with language production and comprehension.

Mixed Dementia

Combination of Pathologies: Mixed dementia involves multiple types of brain pathologies, most commonly Alzheimer's disease and vascular dementia. The coexistence of amyloid plaques, tau tangles, and vascular damage leads to a complex and often more severe cognitive decline.

Complex Symptoms: Symptoms of mixed dementia can vary widely, reflecting the combined effects of the different underlying pathologies. This complexity can make diagnosis and treatment more challenging.

Brain Imaging and Dementia

MRI and CT Scans: Magnetic resonance imaging (MRI) and computed tomography (CT) scans are used to visualize brain structure. These imaging techniques can reveal atrophy, white matter lesions, and other structural changes associated with dementia.

PET Scans: Positron emission tomography (PET) scans can detect amyloid plaques and tau tangles in the brain, aiding in the diagnosis of Alzheimer's disease. PET scans can also measure brain metabolism and blood flow, providing insights into functional changes.

Functional MRI (fMRI): fMRI measures brain activity by detecting changes in blood flow. This technique can show how different brain regions communicate and how this communication is disrupted in dementia.

Dementia affects the brain through a variety of mechanisms, including neuronal death, synaptic dysfunction, inflammation, and specific pathological changes like amyloid plaques, tau tangles, Lewy bodies, and vascular damage. These changes disrupt the brain's structure and function, leading to the cognitive and behavioral symptoms characteristic of dementia. Understanding these processes is crucial for developing effective treatments and providing better care for individuals affected by this condition.

Neurological Basis of Dementia

Understanding the neurological basis of dementia involves examining the specific brain changes and mechanisms that lead to cognitive decline and other symptoms. Dementia is a syndrome caused by various diseases that affect the brain differently. This chapter explores the intricate neurological processes underlying dementia, focusing on key pathologies, neurotransmitter imbalances, and the role of genetic and environmental factors.

Key Pathological Features

Amyloid Plaques: In Alzheimer's disease, the accumulation of amyloid-beta peptides forms plaques between neurons. These plaques interfere with neuronal communication and trigger inflammatory responses that damage brain tissue. The amyloid hypothesis suggests that amyloid-beta aggregation initiates a cascade of events leading to neurodegeneration.

Tau Tangles: Another hallmark of Alzheimer's disease is the formation of neurofibrillary tangles composed of hyperphosphorylated tau protein inside neurons. Tau normally stabilizes microtubules, but when it becomes abnormal, it disrupts cellular transport mechanisms, leading to cell death.

Lewy Bodies: In Lewy body dementia and Parkinson's disease dementia, abnormal aggregates of alpha-synuclein protein, known as Lewy bodies, accumulate within neurons. These inclusions disrupt normal cellular functions and contribute to the loss of dopaminergic neurons, particularly affecting motor and cognitive functions.

Vascular Changes: Vascular dementia results from cerebrovascular disease, including stroke and small vessel disease. Reduced blood flow and oxygen to brain tissues cause ischemic damage and white matter lesions, leading to cognitive deficits. Multiple infarcts or chronic reduced blood supply contribute to widespread brain damage.

Frontotemporal Degeneration: Frontotemporal dementia involves the progressive atrophy of the frontal and temporal lobes. The loss of neurons in these regions affects personality, behavior, and language skills. Pathological changes include tau or TDP-43 protein inclusions, depending on the subtype of frontotemporal dementia.

Neurotransmitter Imbalances

Acetylcholine: Acetylcholine is crucial for learning and memory. In Alzheimer's disease, there is a significant loss of cholinergic neurons, particularly in the basal forebrain, leading to decreased acetylcholine levels. This deficiency contributes to cognitive impairment and memory loss.

Dopamine: Dopamine is essential for motor control, motivation, and reward processing. In Parkinson's disease dementia and Lewy body dementia, dopaminergic neurons in the substantia nigra degenerate, causing motor symptoms and cognitive decline.

Serotonin: Serotonin regulates mood, appetite, and sleep. Changes in serotonin levels and receptor function are observed in various types of dementia, influencing behavioral and psychological symptoms such as depression, aggression, and sleep disturbances.

Glutamate: Glutamate is the primary excitatory neurotransmitter in the brain. Dysregulation of glutamatergic transmission, particularly excessive activation of NMDA receptors, can lead to excitotoxicity and neuronal damage, a process implicated in Alzheimer's disease and other neurodegenerative conditions.

Genetic Factors

APOE4 Gene: The apolipoprotein E (APOE) gene has three common alleles: APOE2, APOE3, and APOE4. The APOE4 allele is a major genetic risk factor for late-onset Alzheimer's disease. Individuals with one or two copies of APOE4 have a significantly increased risk of developing the disease and tend to show symptoms at an earlier age.

PSEN1, PSEN2, and APP Genes: Mutations in these genes are associated with early-onset familial Alzheimer's disease. These mutations lead to abnormal processing of amyloid precursor protein (APP), resulting in increased production of amyloid-beta peptides and plaque formation.

MAPT Gene: Mutations in the microtubule-associated protein tau (MAPT) gene are linked to frontotemporal dementia. These mutations cause tau protein to aggregate abnormally, leading to neuronal damage and brain atrophy.

GRN and C9orf72 Genes: Mutations in the progranulin (GRN) and C9orf72 genes are also associated with frontotemporal dementia. These genetic alterations contribute to neurodegeneration through various mechanisms, including the formation of toxic protein aggregates and impaired cellular functions.

Environmental and Lifestyle Factors

Cardiovascular Health: Cardiovascular risk factors such as hypertension, diabetes, obesity, and smoking are linked to an increased risk of vascular dementia and Alzheimer's disease. Managing these conditions through a healthy lifestyle and medical interventions can help reduce the risk.

Diet and Exercise: A diet rich in antioxidants, healthy fats, and low in refined sugars, such as the Mediterranean diet, is associated with a lower risk of dementia. Regular physical exercise promotes brain health by enhancing blood flow, reducing inflammation, and stimulating neurogenesis.

Cognitive Engagement: Engaging in intellectually stimulating activities throughout life, such as reading, puzzles, and learning new skills, is associated with a reduced risk of dementia. Cognitive reserve, the brain's ability to compensate for damage, is believed to be enhanced by lifelong learning and mental challenges.

Social Connections: Strong social networks and regular social interaction can help protect against cognitive decline. Social engagement stimulates cognitive processes and provides emotional support, both of which are beneficial for brain health.

The neurological basis of dementia involves complex interactions between pathological changes, neurotransmitter imbalances, genetic predispositions, and environmental factors. Understanding these mechanisms is crucial for developing targeted treatments and preventive strategies. By exploring the intricate processes underlying dementia, we can better appreciate the challenges faced by individuals with this condition and work towards improving their quality of life through scientific advancements and supportive care.

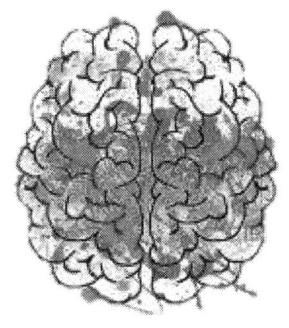

CHAPTER 2:

TYPES OF DEMENTIA

Dementia encompasses a variety of conditions characterized by cognitive decline and impaired memory. Each type has unique causes, symptoms, and progression patterns. This chapter provides an in-depth look at the most common types of dementia, their distinguishing features, and their effects on the brain.

Alzheimer's Disease

Alzheimer's disease is the most common form of dementia, accounting for 60-80% of dementia cases. It is a progressive neurodegenerative disorder that primarily affects older adults, leading to significant cognitive decline, memory loss, and behavioral changes. This chapter delves into the clinical features, pathological mechanisms, risk factors, diagnosis, and treatment of Alzheimer's disease.

Early Symptoms:

Memory Loss: Difficulty remembering recent events or conversations.

Language Problems: Trouble finding the right words or following conversations.

Disorientation: Confusion about time, place, or events.

Difficulty with Complex Tasks: Problems with planning, organizing, and managing finances.

Changes in Mood and Personality: Increased anxiety, depression, irritability, or apathy.

Progression of Symptoms:

Moderate Alzheimer's:

Increased Memory Loss: Forgetting personal history, becoming easily confused.

Difficulty with Daily Activities: Needing help with bathing, dressing, and other personal care.

Behavioral Changes: Wandering, agitation, sleep disturbances, and delusions.

Severe Alzheimer's:

Loss of Independence: Complete dependence on caregivers for daily activities.

Communication Problems: Inability to speak coherently or respond to the environment.

Physical Decline: Difficulty swallowing, incontinence, and immobility.

Pathological Mechanisms

Amyloid Plaques:

Amyloid-beta peptides accumulate and form extracellular plaques, disrupting neuron communication and triggering inflammatory responses. These plaques are a hallmark of Alzheimer's pathology.

Neurofibrillary Tangles:

Abnormal accumulation of hyperphosphorylated tau protein forms tangles within neurons, disrupting the microtubule structure essential for nutrient transport and leading to cell death.

Brain Atrophy:

Significant shrinkage occurs in the hippocampus and cortex, regions crucial for memory and cognitive functions. The extent of atrophy correlates with disease severity.

Chronic Inflammation:

Microglia, the brain's immune cells, become overactive, releasing inflammatory cytokines that contribute to neuronal damage and disease progression.

Risk Factors

Genetic Factors:

APOE4 Allele: The presence of one or two copies of the APOE4 gene variant significantly increases the risk and lowers the age of onset for Alzheimer's.

Familial Alzheimer's Disease: Mutations in genes such as APP, PSEN1, and PSEN2 are linked to early-onset Alzheimer's, leading to amyloid precursor protein misprocessing and increased amyloid-beta production.

Age:

The primary risk factor for Alzheimer's disease, with prevalence doubling every five years after age 65.

Lifestyle and Environmental Factors:

Cardiovascular Health: Hypertension, diabetes, obesity, smoking, and high cholesterol are associated with increased risk.

Diet and Physical Activity: A diet high in saturated fats and lack of physical exercise may contribute to risk, while a Mediterranean diet and regular physical activity are protective.

Education and Cognitive Engagement: Lower levels of formal education and reduced mental stimulation are linked to higher risk, suggesting that cognitive reserve built through lifelong learning may be protective.

Diagnosis

Clinical Assessment:

Detailed patient history, cognitive testing, and assessment of daily functioning. Commonly used tests include the Mini-Mental State Examination (MMSE) and the Montreal Cognitive Assessment (MoCA).

Imaging:

MRI and CT Scans: Used to identify brain atrophy, particularly in the hippocampus and cortex.

PET Scans: Can detect amyloid plaques and tau tangles in the brain, providing a more definitive diagnosis.

Biomarkers:

Cerebrospinal Fluid (CSF) Analysis: Measurement of amyloid-beta and tau levels in CSF can aid in diagnosis.

Blood Tests: Emerging research is exploring blood-based biomarkers for early detection.

Genetic Testing:

Genetic testing for APOE4 and familial Alzheimer's disease mutations may be considered, especially in cases with a strong family history.

Treatment

Pharmacological Treatments:

Cholinesterase Inhibitors: Drugs like donepezil, rivastigmine, and galantamine improve cognitive function by increasing acetylcholine levels in the brain.

NMDA Receptor Antagonists: Memantine helps regulate glutamate activity to improve cognition and daily functioning.

Anti-Amyloid Therapies: Newer treatments aim to reduce amyloid-beta accumulation, such as monoclonal antibodies targeting amyloid plaques.

Non-Pharmacological Interventions:

Cognitive Rehabilitation: Activities designed to improve memory, problem-solving skills, and daily functioning.

Physical Exercise: Regular physical activity can improve overall health and potentially slow cognitive decline.

Social Engagement: Maintaining social connections and participating in group activities can provide emotional support and mental stimulation.

Nutritional Support: A balanced diet, rich in fruits, vegetables, whole grains, and healthy fats, supports brain health.

Support for Caregivers:

Providing education, resources, and support groups to help caregivers manage the challenges of caring for someone with Alzheimer's disease.

Alzheimer's disease is a complex and devastating condition that significantly impacts individuals and their families. Understanding its clinical features, pathological mechanisms, risk factors, and treatment options is crucial for managing the disease and improving the quality of life for those affected. Ongoing research aims to uncover more about the disease's causes and develop more effective treatments, offering hope for the future.

Vascular Dementia

Vascular dementia is the second most common form of dementia, resulting from impaired blood flow to the brain. This condition arises from various vascular issues, including strokes, small vessel disease, and other conditions that damage blood vessels in the brain. This chapter explores the clinical features, underlying mechanisms, risk factors, diagnostic criteria, and treatment options for vascular dementia.

Early Symptoms:

Cognitive Impairment: Difficulty with attention, planning, and problem-solving.

Memory Loss: Less prominent than in Alzheimer's but can occur.

Mood Changes: Depression, apathy, and irritability.

Language Difficulties: Trouble finding words and communicating.

Motor Symptoms: Gait disturbances, slowed movement, and difficulty with coordination.

Progression of Symptoms:

Fluctuating Cognition: Cognitive abilities can vary significantly, with periods of stability followed by sudden declines.

Executive Dysfunction: Difficulty with organizing, making decisions, and handling complex tasks.

Behavioral Changes: Increased anxiety, agitation, and emotional instability.

Physical Symptoms: Muscle weakness, vision problems, and urinary incontinence in advanced stages.

Pathological Mechanisms

Stroke-Related Damage:

Large Vessel Strokes: Major strokes can cause significant brain damage, leading to sudden and severe cognitive decline.

Lacunar Infarcts: Small strokes in the deep brain structures disrupt neural networks, contributing to gradual cognitive deterioration.

Small Vessel Disease:

White Matter Lesions: Chronic high blood pressure and other vascular issues cause damage to the brain's white matter, disrupting the communication between different brain regions.

Microbleeds: Small, asymptomatic bleeds in the brain can accumulate over time, leading to cognitive deficits.

Hypoperfusion:

Reduced blood flow to the brain due to narrowed or blocked arteries causes chronic low oxygen levels, damaging brain cells and contributing to cognitive decline.

Blood-Brain Barrier Dysfunction:

Vascular damage can impair the blood-brain barrier, allowing harmful substances to enter the brain and cause inflammation and neuronal damage.

Risk Factors

Cardiovascular Conditions:

Hypertension: High blood pressure damages blood vessels, increasing the risk of strokes and small vessel disease.

Diabetes: Poorly controlled blood sugar levels lead to vascular damage and increased risk of dementia.

Atherosclerosis: Hardening and narrowing of the arteries reduce blood flow to the brain.

Heart Disease: Conditions like atrial fibrillation increase the risk of blood clots that can cause strokes.

Lifestyle Factors:

Smoking: Increases the risk of cardiovascular disease and subsequent brain damage.

Obesity: Contributes to hypertension, diabetes, and other vascular risk factors.

Physical Inactivity: Lack of exercise worsens cardiovascular health and increases dementia risk.

Unhealthy Diet: Diets high in saturated fats and low in fruits, vegetables, and whole grains contribute to cardiovascular disease.

Genetic Factors:

Family history of stroke or cardiovascular disease can increase the risk of vascular dementia.

Age:

The risk of vascular dementia increases with age, particularly after age 65.

Diagnosis

Clinical Assessment:

Detailed medical history, including cardiovascular health and stroke history.

Cognitive testing to evaluate memory, attention, executive function, and language skills.

Neurological examination to assess motor function, reflexes, and sensory abilities.

Imaging:

MRI and CT Scans: Used to detect strokes, white matter lesions, and other vascular changes in the brain.

Doppler Ultrasound: Assesses blood flow in the neck and brain arteries.

      Vascular dementia is a multifaceted condition resulting from various vascular issues that impair blood flow to the brain. Understanding the clinical features, underlying mechanisms, risk factors, and treatment options is crucial for managing the disease and improving the lives of those affected. Early detection and proactive management of cardiovascular health can help mitigate the impact of vascular dementia and slow its progression.

Lewy Body Dementia

Lewy body dementia (LBD) is a complex and progressive neurodegenerative disorder characterized by the presence of abnormal protein deposits called Lewy bodies in the brain. These deposits disrupt normal brain function, leading to a wide range of cognitive, motor, and behavioral symptoms. LBD includes two related conditions: dementia with Lewy bodies (DLB) and Parkinson's disease dementia (PDD). This chapter explores the clinical features, pathological mechanisms, risk factors, diagnostic criteria, and treatment options for Lewy body dementia.

Clinical Features

Cognitive Symptoms:

Fluctuating Cognition: Cognitive abilities can vary significantly from day to day or even within the same day.

Memory Loss: Similar to Alzheimer's disease, but less prominent in the early stages.

Attention and Executive Function: Difficulties with attention, problem-solving, and planning.

Visual Hallucinations: Vivid and often detailed visual hallucinations are a core feature.

Visuospatial Abilities: Trouble with spatial awareness and navigation.

Motor Symptoms:

Parkinsonism: Motor symptoms such as tremors, muscle rigidity, bradykinesia (slowness of movement), and postural instability.

Gait Abnormalities: Shuffling walk and difficulty with balance.

Behavioral and Psychological Symptoms:

REM Sleep Behavior Disorder (RBD): Acting out dreams during REM sleep, often preceding other symptoms.

Mood Changes: Depression, anxiety, and apathy.

Autonomic Dysfunction: Issues like orthostatic hypotension (sudden drop in blood pressure upon standing), constipation, and urinary incontinence.

Progression of Symptoms:

Early Stage: Mild cognitive impairment, subtle motor symptoms, and REM sleep behavior disorder.

Middle Stage: Increased cognitive decline, more pronounced motor symptoms, and frequent visual hallucinations.

Late Stage: Severe cognitive impairment, significant motor dysfunction, and increased need for assistance with daily activities.

Pathological Mechanisms

Lewy Bodies:

Alpha-Synuclein Deposits: Abnormal accumulations of alpha-synuclein protein form Lewy bodies inside neurons, disrupting cellular function and leading to cell death.

Location: Lewy bodies are found in the cerebral cortex, brainstem, and other brain regions, affecting both cognitive and motor functions.

Neurotransmitter Imbalances:

Dopamine Deficiency: Loss of dopaminergic neurons in the substantia nigra leads to parkinsonian motor symptoms.

Acetylcholine Deficiency: Reduction in cholinergic neurons contributes to cognitive decline and hallucinations.

Brain Atrophy:

Regional Brain Atrophy: Brain imaging often shows atrophy in the frontal and temporal lobes, as well as the brainstem.

Lewy body dementia is a multifaceted and challenging condition that requires a comprehensive approach to diagnosis and management. Understanding its clinical features, underlying mechanisms, risk factors, and treatment options is essential for providing effective care and improving the quality of life for those affected. Ongoing research aims to develop better diagnostic tools and more effective treatments, offering hope for the future in managing this complex disease.

Frontotemporal Dementia

Frontotemporal dementia (FTD) is a group of disorders caused by progressive cell degeneration in the brain's frontal and temporal lobes. These regions are associated with personality, behavior, language, and movement. FTD is often misdiagnosed as a psychiatric disorder or Alzheimer's disease, especially in its early stages, due to overlapping symptoms. This chapter explores the clinical features, pathological mechanisms, risk factors, diagnostic criteria, and treatment options for frontotemporal dementia.

Clinical Features

FTD can be categorized into three primary variants, each with distinct symptoms: behavioral variant (bvFTD), language variant (also known as primary progressive aphasia), and motor variant.

Behavioral Variant (bvFTD):

Personality Changes: Marked alterations in personality and behavior, such as apathy, disinhibition, and loss of empathy.

Impulsivity: Engaging in socially inappropriate behaviors, lack of judgment, and poor impulse control.

Compulsive Behavior: Repetitive actions, such as hoarding or excessive cleaning.

Emotional Blunting: Reduced emotional responsiveness and lack of interest in personal relationships.

Apathy and Inertia: Lack of motivation and difficulty initiating activities.

Language Variant (Primary Progressive Aphasia):

Non-Fluent/Agrammatic Variant (nfvPPA):

Speech Production: Effortful and halting speech, grammatical errors, and difficulty forming sentences.

Agrammatism: Simplified and incorrect grammar usage.

Semantic Variant (svPPA):

Word Comprehension: Loss of understanding of word meanings, naming difficulties, and impaired object recognition.

Fluent Speech: Speech remains fluent but lacks meaning due to semantic deficits.

Logopenic Variant (lvPPA):

Word Finding: Difficulty retrieving words and frequent pauses in speech.

Repetition: Impaired ability to repeat phrases or sentences.

Motor Variant:

Amyotrophic Lateral Sclerosis (ALS): Some individuals with FTD develop ALS, characterized by muscle weakness, atrophy, and spasticity.

Corticobasal Syndrome (CBS): Symptoms include limb rigidity, tremors, and dystonia.

Progressive Supranuclear Palsy (PSP): Difficulty with balance, frequent falls, and eye movement abnormalities.

Pathological Mechanisms

Tau Pathology:

Tau Protein: Abnormal accumulation of tau protein forms tangles within neurons, disrupting cell function and leading to cell death.

MAPT Gene Mutations: Mutations in the MAPT gene, which codes for tau protein, are linked to some cases of FTD.

TDP-43 Proteinopathy:

TDP-43 Protein: Abnormal deposits of TDP-43 protein are found in many cases of FTD, interfering with cellular functions.

GRN Gene Mutations: Mutations in the GRN gene, which affects the production of progranulin, are associated with TDP-43 pathology.

FUS Proteinopathy:

FUS Protein: Abnormal aggregation of FUS protein is less common but also contributes to FTD pathology.

Ubiquitin-Positive Inclusions:

Inclusion Bodies: The presence of ubiquitin-positive inclusions within neurons indicates protein degradation issues.

Risk Factors

Genetic Factors:

Family History: A significant number of FTD cases are familial, suggesting a genetic predisposition.

Specific Gene Mutations: Mutations in genes such as MAPT, GRN, and C9orf72 are strongly associated with FTD.

Age:

FTD typically presents between the ages of 45 and 65, making it one of the leading causes of early-onset dementia.

Sex:

Some forms of FTD show a slight male predominance, but the risk factors do not vary significantly by sex.

Diagnosis

Clinical Assessment:

Detailed patient history, focusing on changes in behavior, personality, and language.

Neurological examination to identify motor symptoms and other neurological deficits.

Cognitive Testing:

Tests designed to assess executive function, language skills, and social cognition.

Imaging:

MRI and CT Scans: To detect atrophy in the frontal and temporal lobes.

PET Scans: To identify changes in brain metabolism that correlate with FTD.

Genetic Testing:

Recommended for patients with a family history of FTD or early-onset dementia to identify specific mutations.

Biomarkers:

Research is ongoing to identify reliable biomarkers in cerebrospinal fluid (CSF) and blood for early detection and diagnosis.

Treatment

Pharmacological Treatments:

Antidepressants: Selective serotonin reuptake inhibitors (SSRIs) may help manage behavioral symptoms such as depression, anxiety, and compulsive behavior.

Antipsychotics: Used cautiously to manage severe behavioral disturbances, though they carry a risk of side effects.

Cholinesterase Inhibitors and Memantine: These Alzheimer's medications are generally not effective in FTD and are used sparingly.

Non-Pharmacological Interventions:

Behavioral Therapy: Tailored interventions to manage specific behavioral problems and improve daily functioning.

Speech and Language Therapy: For patients with primary progressive aphasia, to maintain communication skills and develop alternative communication strategies.

Physical and Occupational Therapy: To address motor symptoms and maintain physical function.

Supportive Care:

Providing education and support for caregivers to manage the complex symptoms of FTD.

Ensuring a safe living environment to accommodate changes in behavior and mobility.

Engaging in social activities and support groups to provide emotional support and reduce isolation.

Lifestyle Modifications:

Healthy Diet: Nutrient-rich diet to support overall brain health.

Regular Exercise: Physical activity to improve overall health and potentially slow disease progression.

Cognitive Engagement: Mental exercises and activities to stimulate cognitive function.

Frontotemporal dementia is a diverse and challenging group of disorders that require a nuanced approach to diagnosis and management. Understanding its clinical features, pathological mechanisms, risk factors, and treatment options is essential for providing effective care and improving the quality of life for patients and their families. Advances in research are crucial for developing better diagnostic tools and more targeted treatments, offering hope for those affected by this complex condition.

Other Forms of Dementia

While Alzheimer's disease, vascular dementia, Lewy body dementia, and frontotemporal dementia are the most well-known types, there are several other forms of dementia that also significantly impact individuals and their families. These less common dementias include mixed dementia, Creutzfeldt-Jakob disease (CJD), normal pressure hydrocephalus (NPH), Huntington's disease, and Wernicke-Korsakoff syndrome. This chapter explores the clinical features, pathological mechanisms, risk factors, diagnostic criteria, and treatment options for these additional types of dementia.

Mixed Dementia

Clinical Features:

Symptoms often overlap with those of Alzheimer's and vascular dementia, including memory loss, confusion, and difficulty with problem-solving.

Varying degrees of cognitive impairment, mood changes, and physical symptoms such as motor dysfunction.

Pathological Mechanisms:

Combination of Alzheimer's pathology (amyloid plaques and tau tangles) and vascular changes (e.g., small strokes, white matter lesions).

Risk Factors:

Age, hypertension, diabetes, and other cardiovascular risk factors.

Diagnosis:

Clinical assessment and imaging studies to identify multiple types of brain pathology.

Treatment:

Combination of treatments used for Alzheimer's and vascular dementia, including medications and lifestyle modifications.

Creutzfeldt-Jakob Disease (CJD)

Clinical Features:

Rapidly progressive dementia, often leading to severe cognitive impairment within months.

Myoclonus (sudden, involuntary muscle jerks), visual disturbances, ataxia (loss of coordination), and other neurological symptoms.

Pathological Mechanisms:

Caused by prion proteins, which induce abnormal folding of normal cellular proteins, leading to brain damage.

Risk Factors:

Sporadic (most common), hereditary, and acquired forms (e.g., through contaminated medical procedures or food).

Diagnosis:

EEG, MRI, and cerebrospinal fluid analysis for 14-3-3 protein. Definitive diagnosis through brain biopsy or autopsy.

Treatment:

No effective cure; treatment focuses on symptom management and supportive care.

Normal Pressure Hydrocephalus (NPH)

Clinical Features:

Triad of symptoms: gait disturbances (shuffling walk, difficulty walking), urinary incontinence, and cognitive impairment.

Pathological Mechanisms:

Accumulation of cerebrospinal fluid (CSF) in the brain's ventricles without increased pressure, leading to ventricular enlargement and compression of brain tissue.

Risk Factors:

Often idiopathic, but can result from head injury, infections, or bleeding in the brain.

Diagnosis:

Clinical assessment, brain imaging (MRI or CT scan), and CSF drainage tests.

Treatment:

Surgical intervention with ventriculoperitoneal shunt to drain excess CSF and alleviate symptoms.

While less common, these additional forms of dementia are equally devastating and require a comprehensive approach to diagnosis and management. Understanding their clinical features, underlying mechanisms, risk factors, and treatment options is crucial for providing effective care and improving the quality of life for those affected. Ongoing research and awareness are essential for advancing our understanding and treatment of these complex conditions.

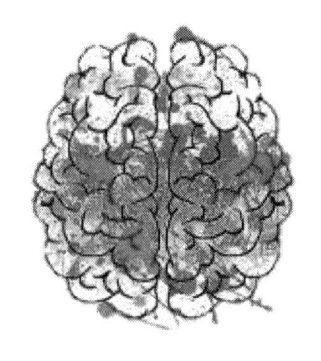

CHAPTER 3:

RISK FACTORS AND CAUSES

Lifestyle and Environmental Factors

The development and progression of dementia are influenced not only by genetic and biological factors but also by lifestyle choices and environmental exposures. Modifiable risk factors related to lifestyle and environment can significantly impact the likelihood of developing dementia, offering opportunities for prevention and intervention. This chapter delves into various lifestyle and environmental factors associated with dementia risk and discusses strategies to mitigate these risks.

Physical Activity

Benefits:

Regular exercise improves cardiovascular health, increases blood flow to the brain, and promotes neurogenesis (the creation of new neurons).

Physical activity helps maintain cognitive function, delay the onset of dementia, and reduce the severity of symptoms.

Recommendations:

Engaging in at least 150 minutes of moderate aerobic exercise, such as brisk walking, per week.

Including strength training exercises at least two days a week to enhance muscle mass and overall physical health.

Diet and Nutrition

Healthy Diet Patterns:

Mediterranean Diet: Rich in fruits, vegetables, whole grains, fish, olive oil, and nuts. Associated with reduced risk of cognitive decline and dementia.

DASH Diet: Focuses on reducing hypertension with high consumption of fruits, vegetables, whole grains, and low-fat dairy products.

Nutritional Factors:

Antioxidants: Foods high in antioxidants, such as berries and leafy greens, help reduce oxidative stress and inflammation in the brain.

Omega-3 Fatty Acids: Found in fatty fish (e.g., salmon, mackerel), omega-3s are essential for brain health and cognitive function.

Vitamins and Minerals: Adequate intake of vitamins (e.g., B vitamins, vitamin D, vitamin E) and minerals (e.g., magnesium) supports cognitive health.

Cognitive Engagement

Mental Stimulation:

Engaging in intellectually stimulating activities (e.g., puzzles, reading, learning new skills) helps build cognitive reserve and maintain brain function.

Lifelong learning and continuous mental challenges are associated with a lower risk of dementia.

Social Engagement:

Maintaining strong social connections and participating in social activities can enhance cognitive function and reduce dementia risk.

Isolation and loneliness are significant risk factors for cognitive decline.

Sleep and Brain Health

Importance of Quality Sleep:

Adequate and restorative sleep is essential for cognitive function and brain health.

Poor sleep quality and sleep disorders (e.g., sleep apnea) are linked to an increased risk of dementia.

Sleep Hygiene Tips:

Maintaining a regular sleep schedule.

Creating a restful sleeping environment.

Avoiding stimulants (e.g., caffeine, nicotine) before bedtime.

Managing stress and anxiety to improve sleep quality.

Chronic Health Conditions

Cardiovascular Health:

Hypertension, diabetes, obesity, and high cholesterol are significant risk factors for dementia.

Managing these conditions through medication, diet, and lifestyle changes can reduce dementia risk.

Mental Health:

Depression and anxiety are associated with an increased risk of cognitive decline and dementia.

Early treatment and management of mental health conditions can improve cognitive outcomes.

Substance Use

Alcohol Consumption:

Excessive alcohol use is a known risk factor for cognitive decline and dementia (e.g., alcohol-related dementia, Wernicke-Korsakoff syndrome).

Moderate alcohol consumption, particularly wine, may have a protective effect, though this is still under investigation.

Smoking:

Smoking is linked to vascular damage and increased risk of vascular dementia and Alzheimer's disease.

Quitting smoking at any age can improve brain health and reduce dementia risk.

Environmental Factors

Pollution:

Exposure to air pollution, heavy metals, and toxic chemicals is associated with an increased risk of cognitive impairment and dementia.

Policies and practices that reduce environmental pollutants can contribute to better brain health.

Head Injuries:

Traumatic brain injury (TBI) is a significant risk factor for dementia, particularly chronic traumatic encephalopathy (CTE).

Wearing protective gear during sports and activities, and preventing falls in older adults can reduce the risk of head injuries.

 Lifestyle and environmental factors play a crucial role in the development and progression of dementia. By adopting healthy lifestyle habits, managing chronic health conditions, and reducing exposure to environmental risks, individuals can significantly lower their risk of cognitive decline and dementia. Public health initiatives and policies aimed at promoting brain health and preventing dementia are essential for addressing the growing global impact of this condition.

Comorbid Conditions

Dementia often coexists with other medical conditions, which can complicate diagnosis, treatment, and care. Understanding these comorbid conditions is crucial for comprehensive management of individuals with dementia, as they can exacerbate cognitive symptoms and impact the overall quality of life. This chapter explores the common comorbidities associated with dementia, their effects on patients, and strategies for managing these conditions.

Cardiovascular Diseases

Hypertension:

Impact on Dementia: High blood pressure is a significant risk factor for both vascular dementia and Alzheimer's disease. It can lead to small vessel disease, white matter lesions, and brain infarcts.

Management: Controlling blood pressure through lifestyle changes, medications, and regular monitoring can reduce the risk of cognitive decline.

Heart Disease:

Impact on Dementia: Conditions such as coronary artery disease and heart failure reduce cerebral blood flow, contributing to cognitive impairment.

Management: Managing heart disease with medications, lifestyle modifications, and possibly surgical interventions can improve cognitive outcomes.

Stroke:

Impact on Dementia: Strokes can cause immediate and long-term cognitive deficits, and individuals who have had a stroke are at a higher risk of developing dementia.

Management: Preventing strokes through anticoagulants, antiplatelet agents, and controlling risk factors like hypertension and diabetes is critical.

Metabolic Disorders

Diabetes:

Impact on Dementia: Diabetes is associated with an increased risk of Alzheimer's disease and vascular dementia. Poor glycemic control can lead to neurodegenerative changes and cerebrovascular damage.

Management: Maintaining blood sugar levels through diet, exercise, medications, and regular monitoring can help mitigate cognitive decline.

Hyperlipidemia:

Impact on Dementia: Elevated cholesterol levels are linked to an increased risk of vascular dementia and Alzheimer's disease.

Management: Using statins and other lipid-lowering agents, along with lifestyle changes, can improve cardiovascular health and potentially reduce dementia risk.

Psychiatric Disorders

Depression:

Impact on Dementia: Depression is both a risk factor and a common comorbidity in dementia, potentially worsening cognitive symptoms and decreasing the quality of life.

Management: Treating depression with antidepressants, psychotherapy, and lifestyle interventions can improve mood and cognitive function.

Anxiety:

Impact on Dementia: Anxiety disorders can exacerbate cognitive symptoms and increase stress, negatively impacting individuals with dementia.

Management: Anti-anxiety medications, counseling, and stress management techniques can help reduce anxiety and improve overall well-being.

Psychosis:

Impact on Dementia: Hallucinations and delusions are common in certain types of dementia, such as Lewy body dementia and Alzheimer's disease, and can lead to significant distress.

Management: Antipsychotic medications, used cautiously, along with non-pharmacological approaches, can manage psychotic symptoms.

Respiratory Conditions

Chronic Obstructive Pulmonary Disease (COPD):

Impact on Dementia: COPD can lead to hypoxia and hypercapnia, both of which can impair cognitive function.

Management: Optimizing respiratory function through medications, oxygen therapy, and pulmonary rehabilitation can improve cognitive outcomes.

Sleep Apnea:

Impact on Dementia: Obstructive sleep apnea (OSA) is associated with cognitive decline due to intermittent hypoxia and sleep fragmentation.

Management: Continuous positive airway pressure (CPAP) therapy, weight management, and avoiding alcohol can improve sleep quality and cognitive function.

Neurological Disorders

Parkinson's Disease:

Impact on Dementia: Many individuals with Parkinson's disease develop cognitive impairment, known as Parkinson's disease dementia (PDD).

Management: Medications like levodopa can manage motor symptoms, while cholinesterase inhibitors may help with cognitive symptoms.

Epilepsy:

Impact on Dementia: Seizures can cause transient or permanent cognitive impairments, particularly in older adults.

Management: Antiepileptic drugs (AEDs) should be carefully selected to avoid cognitive side effects while effectively controlling seizures.

Autoimmune and Inflammatory Conditions

Rheumatoid Arthritis:

Impact on Dementia: Chronic inflammation associated with rheumatoid arthritis may contribute to cognitive decline.

Management: Anti-inflammatory medications and disease-modifying antirheumatic drugs (DMARDs) can help manage rheumatoid arthritis and potentially reduce dementia risk.

Systemic Lupus Erythematosus (SLE):

Impact on Dementia: Neuropsychiatric lupus can cause cognitive dysfunction, often referred to as lupus brain fog.

Management: Managing lupus with immunosuppressive therapies and corticosteroids can help control symptoms and improve cognitive function.

Cancer and Cancer Treatment

Cancer:

Impact on Dementia: Certain cancers and cancer treatments (e.g., chemotherapy) can lead to cognitive deficits known as "chemo brain."

Management: Supportive therapies, cognitive rehabilitation, and managing cancer-related fatigue can improve cognitive symptoms.

Paraneoplastic Syndromes:

Impact on Dementia: These syndromes, caused by the immune response to cancer, can lead to significant neurological and cognitive impairment.

Management: Treating the underlying cancer and using immunosuppressive therapies can help manage symptoms.

Infectious Diseases

HIV/AIDS:

Impact on Dementia: HIV-associated neurocognitive disorder (HAND) includes a spectrum of cognitive impairments resulting from the direct effects of HIV on the brain.

Management: Antiretroviral therapy (ART) can significantly reduce the risk and severity of HAND.

Syphilis:

Impact on Dementia: Neurosyphilis, resulting from untreated syphilis infection, can cause cognitive decline and dementia-like symptoms.

Management: Early diagnosis and treatment with antibiotics can prevent or reverse cognitive symptoms.

Managing comorbid conditions in individuals with dementia is crucial for improving their overall health, cognitive function, and quality of life. A multidisciplinary approach that addresses both dementia and its comorbidities can provide comprehensive care, reduce complications, and enhance patient outcomes. Regular monitoring, personalized treatment plans, and supportive interventions are essential for addressing the complex needs of individuals with dementia and their caregivers.

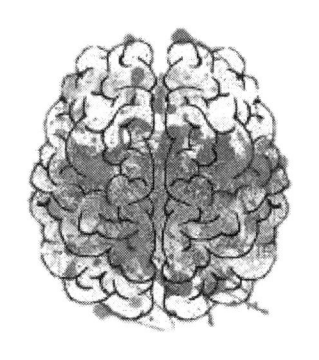

CHAPTER 4:

DIAGNOSIS AND EARLY DETECTION OF DEMENTIA

Diagnosing dementia involves a comprehensive assessment of cognitive, functional, and behavioral changes, along with identifying potential underlying causes. Early detection is crucial for timely intervention and improved management of the condition. This chapter explores the diagnostic process, screening tools, clinical assessments, and emerging technologies used in the diagnosis and early detection of dementia.

Symptoms and Early Signs

Recognizing the early signs and symptoms of dementia is vital for timely diagnosis, intervention, and management. Dementia encompasses a range of cognitive, behavioral, and psychological changes that progressively impair daily functioning. This chapter outlines the common symptoms and early signs observed in individuals with dementia across various types, emphasizing the importance of early detection and evaluation.

Cognitive Symptoms

Memory Loss:

Short-Term Memory: Forgetting recent events, appointments, or conversations.

Long-Term Memory: Difficulty recalling past memories and details about one's life history.

Difficulty with Planning and Organization:

Challenges in following a sequence of steps (e.g., cooking a meal) or planning activities for the day.

Misplacing items or struggling to organize tasks at home or work.

Impaired Judgment and Decision-Making:

Making poor decisions, especially in financial matters or judgment of safety.

Difficulty weighing risks and benefits or understanding consequences.

Language and Communication Problems:

Word Finding Difficulty: Struggling to find the right words or names of familiar objects.

Aphasia: Difficulty understanding or producing speech, including grammatical errors or fluent but nonsensical speech.

Spatial and Visual Disorientation:

Getting lost in familiar places or difficulty following directions.

Problems with depth perception or visual-spatial relationships (e.g., judging distances).

Behavioral and Psychological Symptoms

Changes in Mood and Personality:

Mood swings, irritability, or agitation without apparent cause.

Withdrawal from social activities or loss of interest in hobbies.

Disinhibition and Impulsivity:

Behaving in socially inappropriate ways, such as making rude comments or disregarding personal boundaries.

Acting impulsively without considering consequences.

Apathy and Loss of Initiative:

Lack of motivation or interest in activities previously enjoyed.

Reduced engagement in social interactions or neglect of personal care.

Psychiatric Symptoms:

Depression: Persistent sadness, feelings of hopelessness, or loss of interest in activities.

Anxiety: Excessive worry, restlessness, or fearfulness about everyday situations.

Functional Impairments

Difficulties with Activities of Daily Living (ADLs):

Challenges in performing self-care tasks such as bathing, dressing, or grooming.

Needing assistance with household chores or managing finances.

Work and Social Impairments:

Decline in work performance, such as making mistakes or difficulty completing tasks.

Social withdrawal or difficulty maintaining relationships due to communication or behavioral changes.

Progressive Nature of Symptoms

Gradual Onset and Progression:

Early symptoms may be subtle and easily overlooked, progressing over months to years.

Symptoms worsen over time, leading to significant impairment in daily functioning and independence.

Variability Across Dementia Types

Alzheimer's Disease:

Early symptoms often involve memory loss, particularly recent events or conversations.

Progresses to include language difficulties, confusion, and disorientation.

Vascular Dementia:

Symptoms may occur suddenly after a stroke or gradually due to multiple small strokes.

Cognitive impairments vary based on the location and severity of vascular damage.

Lewy Body Dementia:

Visual hallucinations, fluctuating cognition, and Parkinsonism (e.g., tremors, stiffness) are early features.

Sleep disturbances and sensitivity to medications are common.

Frontotemporal Dementia:

Changes in behavior, personality, and language skills predominate early.

Memory loss may be less prominent compared to alterations in social conduct or speech.

Recognizing Early Signs

Observation and Documentation:

Caregivers, family members, or healthcare providers should note changes in behavior, cognition, and daily function.

Keeping a journal of symptoms can aid in tracking progression and informing medical evaluations.

Seeking Medical Evaluation:

Consultation with a healthcare professional, such as a neurologist or geriatrician, for comprehensive assessment and diagnosis.

Early intervention allows for timely treatment, support services, and planning for future care needs.

Early recognition of symptoms and signs of dementia is essential for initiating appropriate diagnostic evaluations and interventions. Awareness of cognitive, behavioral, and functional changes enables individuals, caregivers, and healthcare providers to address concerns promptly and plan for optimal management of dementia. Ongoing research and public education are critical for enhancing early detection efforts and improving outcomes for individuals affected by this progressive condition.

Diagnostic Procedures

Accurate diagnosis of dementia involves a systematic approach that integrates clinical evaluations, cognitive assessments, imaging studies, and laboratory tests. This chapter provides an overview of the diagnostic procedures used to evaluate individuals suspected of having dementia, emphasizing the importance of comprehensive assessment and differential diagnosis.

Clinical Evaluation

History Taking:

Detailed history from the patient and caregivers to identify onset, progression, and nature of cognitive symptoms.

Inquiring about medical history, medications, family history of dementia, and lifestyle factors.

Physical Examination:

Assessment of general health, neurological function, and evaluation for signs of underlying conditions contributing to cognitive decline.

Examination of vital signs, cardiovascular health, and neurological abnormalities (e.g., gait, reflexes).

Cognitive Assessments

Mini-Mental State Examination (MMSE):

Brief screening tool assessing orientation, memory, attention, language, and visuospatial abilities.

Scores below a certain threshold indicate cognitive impairment warranting further evaluation.

Montreal Cognitive Assessment (MoCA):

Assess broader cognitive domains, including executive function, and is sensitive to mild cognitive impairment (MCI) and early dementia.

Clock Drawing Test:

Assesses visuospatial abilities and executive function by asking individuals to draw a clock face showing a specific time.

Neuropsychological Testing

Comprehensive Neuropsychological Battery:

Evaluates multiple cognitive domains (e.g., memory, language, executive function) through standardized tests.

Provides detailed assessment of strengths and weaknesses in cognitive abilities.

Imaging Studies

Structural Imaging:

MRI (Magnetic Resonance Imaging): Provides detailed images of brain structure, detecting atrophy, lesions, and changes in specific regions (e.g., hippocampus).

CT (Computed Tomography): Used to rule out other causes of cognitive impairment, such as tumors or strokes.

Functional Imaging:

PET (Positron Emission Tomography): Measures brain metabolism and detects changes in glucose uptake or amyloid deposition (used in Alzheimer's diagnosis).

SPECT (Single Photon Emission Computed Tomography): Assesses regional cerebral blood flow, beneficial in diagnosing vascular dementia.

Biomarker Testing

Cerebrospinal Fluid (CSF) Analysis:

Examination of CSF biomarkers such as amyloid beta and tau proteins to assess Alzheimer's disease pathology.

Used in research and specialized diagnostic settings.

Blood Tests:

Rule out reversible causes of cognitive impairment (e.g., vitamin deficiencies, thyroid dysfunction).

Genetic testing for familial forms of dementia (e.g., Alzheimer's disease, frontotemporal dementia).

Diagnosing dementia requires a comprehensive approach that includes clinical evaluation, cognitive assessments, imaging studies, biomarker testing, and genetic analysis. Early and accurate diagnosis allows for timely intervention, appropriate management strategies, and support for individuals and their families affected by dementia. Ongoing research and advances in diagnostic technologies continue to improve diagnostic accuracy and pave the way for personalized approaches to dementia care.

Importance of Early Diagnosis

Early diagnosis of dementia is crucial for several reasons, impacting both individuals affected by the condition and their caregivers. Recognizing and evaluating symptoms promptly can lead to improved management strategies, better outcomes, and enhanced quality of life.

Timely Intervention and Treatment

Access to Therapies:

Early diagnosis facilitates timely initiation of pharmacological treatments (e.g., cholinesterase inhibitors, memantine) that may slow cognitive decline and manage symptoms.

Allows for participation in clinical trials testing new therapies and interventions aimed at delaying disease progression.

Non-pharmacological Interventions:

Early identification enables individuals and families to access non-pharmacological interventions, such as cognitive stimulation programs, occupational therapy, and caregiver support services.

Provides opportunities for lifestyle modifications (e.g., diet, exercise, cognitive training) that can improve overall brain health and delay functional decline.

Care Planning and Decision Making

Advance Care Planning:

Allows individuals to participate in decisions regarding their future care preferences, financial planning, and legal matters (e.g., power of attorney, living will).

Reduces burden on caregivers by clarifying preferences and ensuring alignment with individual values and wishes.

Caregiver Support and Education:

Early diagnosis provides caregivers with the opportunity to seek education, training, and support services tailored to managing dementia-related challenges.

Enhances caregiver preparedness, reduces stress, and promotes resilience in managing caregiving responsibilities.

Safety and Risk Management

Driving and Safety Precautions:

Allows for early implementation of safety measures, including evaluation of driving abilities and making necessary adjustments to ensure safety on the road.

Addresses safety risks associated with cognitive impairments, such as preventing falls and managing medication adherence.

Financial and Legal Planning:

Early diagnosis enables individuals and families to address financial planning, including managing finances, estate planning, and accessing social support programs.

Mitigates risks of financial exploitation and ensures legal protections are in place to safeguard assets and decision-making authority.

Psychological and Emotional Well-being

Reducing Anxiety and Uncertainty:

Early diagnosis provides clarity and validation of symptoms, reducing anxiety associated with uncertainty and misinterpretation of cognitive changes.

Facilitates emotional adjustment and adaptation to the diagnosis, allowing individuals and families to seek emotional support and coping strategies.

Early diagnosis of dementia is instrumental in improving outcomes for individuals, families, and society at large. It facilitates timely access to treatments and interventions, supports care planning and decision-making, enhances safety and risk management, promotes psychological well-being, contributes to research advancements, and informs public health strategies. By prioritizing early detection and intervention, healthcare systems can optimize dementia care, improve quality of life, and ultimately work towards reducing the global impact of this complex condition.

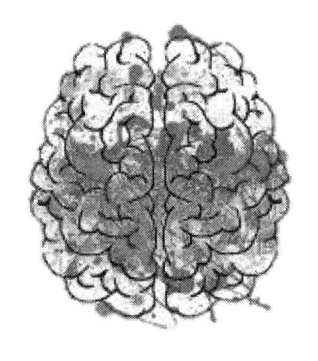

CHAPTER 5:

CARING FOR SOMEONE WITH DEMENTIA

Caring for someone with dementia requires patience, understanding, and a compassionate approach. This chapter explores essential aspects of caregiving, including practical strategies, emotional support, and resources for caregivers to provide effective and empathetic care to individuals with dementia.

Roles and Responsibilities of Caregivers

Caring for someone with dementia involves fulfilling a range of roles and responsibilities to ensure their physical, emotional, and social well-being. This chapter outlines the essential roles caregivers play in providing compassionate and effective care to individuals with dementia, emphasizing the diverse tasks and challenges caregivers may encounter.

Primary Roles of Caregivers

1. Personal Care Assistance:

Assisting with Activities of Daily Living (ADLs): Help with tasks such as bathing, dressing, grooming, toileting, and feeding as needed.

Mobility Support: Provide assistance with walking, transferring between chairs or beds, and ensuring safety during movement.

2. Medication Management:

Administering Medications: Ensure medications are taken as prescribed, manage pill schedules, and monitor for side effects or changes in condition.

Tracking and Refilling Prescriptions: Maintain records of medications, refill prescriptions, and communicate with healthcare providers as necessary.

3. Daily Living Support:

Meal Preparation: Plan and prepare nutritious meals that meet dietary needs and preferences, ensuring adequate nutrition and hydration.

Household Management: Assist with household chores such as cleaning, laundry, and organizing living spaces to maintain a safe and comfortable environment.

4. Cognitive and Emotional Support:

Engaging Activities: Plan and participate in activities that stimulate cognitive function, memory recall, and social interaction.

Emotional Support: Provide companionship, empathy, and reassurance to alleviate anxiety, confusion, or emotional distress.

Responsibilities of Caregivers

1. Monitoring Health and Well-being:

Observation and Reporting: Monitor changes in physical health, cognitive function, and behavior, and report concerns to healthcare professionals.

Vital Signs Monitoring: Track vital signs such as blood pressure, temperature, and pulse to identify any abnormalities or health issues.

2. Communication and Advocacy:

Healthcare Coordination: Facilitate communication between healthcare providers, coordinate medical appointments, and convey information about the individual's condition and needs.

Advocacy: Advocate for the individual's rights, preferences, and quality of care within healthcare settings and community resources.

3. Care Planning and Decision Making:

Care Plan Development: Collaborate with healthcare teams to develop and adjust care plans that address the individual's evolving needs and goals.

Advance Care Planning: Discuss and document preferences for future medical care, end-of-life decisions, and legal matters such as power of attorney.

4. Family and Social Support:

Family Communication: Keep family members informed about the individual's condition, care needs, and updates on their well-being.

Social Engagement: Encourage social interactions, visits from friends and family, and participation in community activities to promote social connection and reduce isolation.

Emotional and Practical Challenges

1. Emotional Resilience:

Stress Management: Practice self-care strategies such as exercise, relaxation techniques, and seeking emotional support from friends, support groups, or counseling.

Coping with Grief and Loss: Navigate feelings of grief and loss associated with changes in the individual's abilities, roles, and relationships.

2. Financial and Legal Responsibilities:

Financial Management: Manage finances, budgeting, and handling financial transactions on behalf of the individual, ensuring financial stability and security.

Legal Guidance: Seek legal advice to address legal matters such as estate planning, guardianship, and executing legal documents (e.g., wills, trusts).

Collaboration and Community Resources

1. Healthcare Collaboration:

Team Approach: Work collaboratively with healthcare professionals, including doctors, nurses, therapists, and social workers, to coordinate comprehensive care.

Educational Opportunities: Attend caregiver education programs, workshops, and training sessions to enhance caregiving skills and knowledge.

2. Utilizing Community Resources:

Respite Care Services: Arrange respite care to provide temporary relief and prevent caregiver burnout, allowing time for rest and rejuvenation.

Support Services: Access community resources such as dementia support groups, caregiver support networks, and home health services for additional assistance and guidance.

Caregivers play a vital role in supporting individuals with dementia by providing personalized care, advocacy, emotional support, and managing day-to-day responsibilities. By embracing their roles with compassion, resilience, and dedication, caregivers can enhance the quality of life for their loved ones while navigating the challenges and complexities associated with dementia caregiving. Collaboration with healthcare professionals and utilization of available resources are essential in providing holistic care and ensuring the well-being of both caregivers and individuals living with dementia.

Daily Care Routines

Establishing a structured daily care routine is crucial for individuals with dementia to provide stability, promote independence, and enhance their overall well-being. This chapter outlines a comprehensive daily care routine tailored to meet the unique needs and challenges faced by individuals living with dementia.

Morning Routine

1. Wake-Up and Personal Hygiene:

Gently wake the individual at a consistent time each day to establish a routine.

Assist with morning hygiene tasks such as brushing teeth, washing face, and toileting needs.

2. Dressing and Grooming:

Lay out clothing choices in advance to simplify decision-making.

Provide assistance as needed with dressing, ensuring clothing is comfortable and weather-appropriate.

3. Breakfast and Medication:

Prepare a nutritious breakfast that aligns with dietary preferences and restrictions.

Administer medications as prescribed, ensuring adherence to medication schedules.

Daytime Activities

1. Structured Activities:

Plan engaging activities that stimulate cognitive function and physical activity, such as puzzles, arts and crafts, or gentle exercises.

Encourage participation in hobbies or interests that the individual enjoys.

2. Meal Preparation and Nutrition:

Offer balanced meals and snacks throughout the day, incorporating fruits, vegetables, whole grains, and lean proteins.

Ensure adequate hydration by providing water and other beverages regularly.

3. Cognitive Stimulation:

Incorporate memory games, storytelling, or reminiscence activities to promote cognitive stimulation and memory recall.

Use tools like memory aids or calendars to reinforce daily routines and important events.

Afternoon and Evening Routine

1. Rest and Relaxation:

Provide opportunities for rest or quiet time in the afternoon to prevent fatigue.

Encourage relaxation techniques such as listening to calming music or guided meditation.

2. Social Interaction:

Facilitate social engagement through visits from family and friends, phone calls, or virtual interactions.

Attend community activities or support groups tailored for individuals with dementia.

3. Dinner and Evening Preparations:

Prepare a nutritious dinner that is easy to chew and swallow, if needed.

Assist with evening hygiene routines such as bathing or showering, and dressing in comfortable sleepwear.

Nighttime Routine

1. Bedtime Preparations:

Establish a calming bedtime routine with consistent activities such as reading a book or listening to soothing music.

Ensure the bedroom environment is conducive to sleep, adjusting lighting and temperature as necessary.

2. Medication Administration:

Administer any nighttime medications prescribed by healthcare providers.

Monitor for any discomfort or sleep disturbances, providing comfort and reassurance.

3. Safety Checks:

Conduct safety checks to prevent falls or accidents during the night, ensuring pathways are clear and night lights are accessible.

Consider using assistive devices such as bed rails or motion sensors to enhance safety.

Tips for Implementing a Successful Daily Routine

1. Flexibility and Patience:

Adapt the routine based on the individual's preferences, abilities, and current mood.

Be patient and allow extra time for tasks, understanding that some days may be more challenging than others.

2. Consistency and Predictability:

Maintain consistency in daily activities, meal times, and sleep schedules to establish a sense of stability.

Use visual cues, calendars, or clocks to reinforce the sequence of daily events and transitions.

3. Communication and Empathy:

Communicate clearly and positively, using gentle prompts and encouragement throughout the day.

Approach caregiving with empathy and understanding, respecting the individual's dignity and autonomy.

A well-structured daily care routine provides individuals with dementia a sense of security, independence, and familiarity, promoting overall well-being and quality of life. By incorporating personalized activities, nutritious meals, cognitive stimulation, and emotional support into daily routines, caregivers can create a nurturing environment that enhances the individual's comfort and satisfaction. Flexibility, patience, and ongoing communication are key in adapting the routine to meet evolving needs and preferences, ensuring a positive caregiving experience for both the individual with dementia and their caregivers.

Managing Stress and Caregiver Burnout

Caring for a loved one with dementia can be rewarding, but it also comes with significant challenges that can lead to stress and caregiver burnout. This chapter explores effective strategies and practical tips for caregivers to manage stress, maintain their well-being, and prevent burnout while providing compassionate care to individuals with dementia.

Understanding Stress and Burnout

1. Recognizing Signs of Stress:

Physical: Fatigue, headaches, sleep disturbances, and changes in appetite.

Emotional: Anxiety, irritability, sadness, feelings of guilt or helplessness.

Behavioral: Withdrawal from activities, social isolation, neglecting personal responsibilities.

2. Impact of Caregiver Burnout:

Reduced quality of care for the individual with dementia due to emotional and physical exhaustion.

Increased risk of health problems, depression, and caregiver resentment or strain in relationships.

Strategies for Managing Stress

1. Self-Care and Personal Well-being:

Prioritize Self-Care: Make time for activities that recharge and relax you, such as exercise, hobbies, reading, or spending time outdoors.

Maintain a Healthy Lifestyle: Eat nutritious meals, stay hydrated, and get enough rest to sustain physical and emotional resilience.

Seek Support: Connect with friends, family, or support groups to share experiences, seek advice, and receive emotional support.

2. Time Management and Setting Boundaries:

Establish Realistic Expectations: Recognize and accept that caregiving has its limitations; prioritize tasks and delegate responsibilities when possible.

Set Boundaries: Learn to say no to additional commitments that may overwhelm you, and communicate your needs clearly to family members and friends.

3. Seek Respite and Support Services:

Take Breaks: Arrange regular respite care to give yourself time away from caregiving responsibilities, allowing for relaxation and rejuvenation.

Utilize Support Resources: Access community resources, such as adult day programs or in-home care services, to provide temporary relief and assistance.

Coping Strategies for Emotional Well-being

1. Practice Stress Reduction Techniques:

Deep Breathing and Relaxation: Engage in deep breathing exercises, meditation, or yoga to calm the mind and reduce stress levels.

Mindfulness: Practice mindfulness techniques to stay present in the moment and manage negative thoughts or worries.

2. Maintain Positive Relationships:

Stay Connected: Nurture relationships with friends and family members who provide emotional support and understanding.

Join Support Groups: Participate in caregiver support groups or online forums to connect with others facing similar challenges and share coping strategies.

Professional Support and Caregiver Education

1. Educate Yourself About Dementia:

Knowledge Empowers: Learn about the specific type of dementia affecting your loved one, its symptoms, progression, and effective caregiving strategies.

Attend Workshops and Training: Take advantage of caregiver education programs, workshops, or online courses to enhance your caregiving skills and confidence.

2. Professional Counseling and Therapy:

Seek Professional Help: Consider therapy or counseling sessions to process emotions, address caregiver stress, and develop coping mechanisms.

Consult Healthcare Providers: Discuss your concerns with healthcare professionals to explore options for managing stress and improving your well-being.

Managing stress and preventing caregiver burnout are essential for sustaining compassionate and effective care for individuals with dementia. By prioritizing self-care, seeking support from others, and accessing respite and professional services, caregivers can maintain their own well-being while providing high-quality care. Understanding the signs of stress, practicing stress management techniques, and planning for future care needs are crucial steps in promoting resilience and ensuring a positive caregiving experience for both caregivers and their loved ones with dementia.

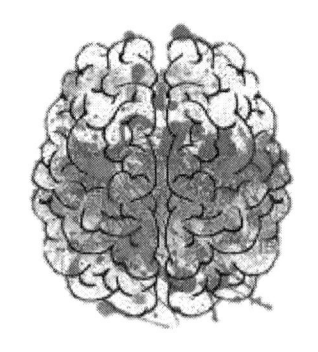

CHAPTER 6:

COMMINICATION STRATEGIES

Effective communication is essential when caring for someone with dementia. As cognitive abilities decline, individuals may experience challenges in expressing themselves and understanding others. This chapter explores practical communication strategies and techniques tailored to enhance understanding, minimize frustration, and promote meaningful interactions with individuals living with dementia.

Effective Communication Techniques

Effective communication is crucial for maintaining meaningful connections and providing compassionate care to individuals with dementia. As cognitive abilities decline, communication strategies need to be adapted to enhance understanding, reduce frustration, and support overall well-being. This chapter explores practical and effective communication techniques that caregivers can employ in their interactions with individuals living with dementia.

1. Simplify Language and Speak Clearly:

Use simple and concise sentences, avoiding complex language or abstract concepts.

Break down instructions or information into smaller, manageable parts to facilitate understanding.

2. Maintain a Calm and Respectful Tone:

Speak in a gentle, calm, and reassuring tone to convey warmth and support.

Avoid speaking loudly or using a condescending tone, which can cause agitation or confusion.

3. Use Nonverbal Communication:

Facial Expressions and Eye Contact: Maintain eye contact and use facial expressions to convey emotions and intentions.

Gestures and Body Language: Use gestures, nods, and physical cues to reinforce verbal messages and aid comprehension.

4. Provide Visual Cues and Prompts:

Use visual aids such as pictures, written notes, or objects to supplement verbal communication.

Point to or show items related to the topic of conversation to enhance understanding and memory recall.

5. Encourage and Validate Responses:

Allow ample time for the individual to process information and formulate responses.

Validate their feelings and responses, even if they may seem repetitive or unrelated, to show empathy and understanding.

6. Focus on Feelings and Emotions:

Acknowledge and respond to the emotions expressed by the individual, focusing on their feelings rather than factual details.

Use empathetic responses to validate their experiences and provide comfort (e.g., "I can see this is frustrating for you").

7. Avoid Arguing or Correcting:

Refrain from arguing or correcting factual inaccuracies, as this can lead to frustration and escalate the situation.

Instead, redirect the conversation to a different topic or activity if disagreements arise.

8. Use Positive Reinforcement and Encouragement:

Offer praise and positive reinforcement for efforts made in communication or completing tasks.

Celebrate achievements and milestones, no matter how small, to boost their confidence and morale.

9. Be Patient and Flexible:

Practice patience and maintain a flexible approach to communication, adapting to the individual's changing abilities and needs.

Take breaks as needed to manage your own emotions and return to the conversation with a calm demeanor.

10. Create a Supportive Environment:

Choose quiet, well-lit spaces for conversations to minimize distractions and improve focus.

Ensure the individual feels comfortable and respected, promoting a supportive and nurturing environment for communication.

11. Listen Actively and Respond Empathetically:

Practice active listening by paying attention to verbal and nonverbal cues, and responding appropriately.

Show empathy and understanding through your responses, demonstrating that you are present and attentive to their needs.

12. Seek Professional Guidance and Support:

Consult healthcare professionals, speech therapists, or dementia specialists for guidance on effective communication techniques.

Attend caregiver support groups or workshops to learn new strategies and share experiences with other caregivers.

By employing these effective communication techniques, caregivers can foster meaningful connections, reduce misunderstandings, and enhance the quality of life for individuals living with dementia. Patience, empathy, and adaptability are essential in navigating communication challenges and promoting a positive caregiving experience. Continuous learning and collaboration with healthcare professionals and support networks can further strengthen caregivers' abilities to communicate effectively and provide compassionate care to their loved ones with dementia.

Understanding Behavioral Changes

Behavioral changes are common in individuals with dementia and can present challenges for both the person affected and their caregivers. This chapter explores the causes, types, and strategies for understanding and managing behavioral changes associated with dementia.

Causes of Behavioral Changes

1. Neurological Changes:

Brain Damage: Dementia causes progressive damage to brain cells, affecting cognitive function and behavior.

Chemical Imbalances: Changes in brain chemistry can influence mood, emotions, and behavior.

2. Physical Health Issues:

Pain or Discomfort: Individuals with dementia may have difficulty expressing physical discomfort, leading to changes in behavior.

Illness or Infections: Medical conditions or infections can exacerbate behavioral symptoms.

3. Environmental Factors:

Stress or Overstimulation: Loud noises, crowded spaces, or unfamiliar environments can trigger agitation or anxiety.

Lack of Routine: Disruptions in daily routines or changes in caregiving practices can contribute to behavioral changes.

Types of Behavioral Changes

1. Agitation and Aggression:

Restlessness: Pacing, fidgeting, or inability to sit still.

Verbal or Physical Aggression: Outbursts, shouting, or physical confrontations.

2. Anxiety and Depression:

Worry or Fearfulness: Constant worrying, suspicion, or paranoia.

Sadness or Hopelessness: Tearfulness, withdrawal from activities, or loss of interest.

3. Sundowning Syndrome:

Increased Confusion: Worsening of symptoms in the late afternoon or evening.

Restlessness or Agitation: Disorientation, wandering, or difficulty sleeping.

4. Repetitive Behaviors:

Repetition: Repeating questions, phrases, or activities.

Pacing or Rocking: Engaging in repetitive movements as a coping mechanism.

5. Hallucinations or Delusions:

Perceptual Changes: Seeing, hearing, or feeling things that are not present (hallucinations).

False Beliefs: Holding onto false or irrational beliefs (delusions).

Strategies for Understanding and Managing Behavioral Changes

1. Identify Triggers and Patterns:

Observe and Document: Keep track of behaviors, triggers, and environmental factors that precede or exacerbate changes.

Consult Healthcare Professionals: Seek guidance from doctors, nurses, or specialists to understand underlying causes and develop management strategies.

2. Create a Calming Environment:

Reduce Stimuli: Minimize noise, distractions, and clutter in the environment.

Establish Routines: Maintain predictable daily routines to provide structure and reduce anxiety.

3. Validate Feelings and Provide Reassurance:

Empathize: Acknowledge the person's feelings and respond with understanding and reassurance.

Redirect Attention: Distract the individual with a comforting activity or topic of conversation to alleviate distress.

4. Communication Strategies:

Use Clear and Simple Language: Speak calmly and use straightforward sentences to facilitate understanding.

Nonverbal Cues: Use gestures, facial expressions, and touch to convey empathy and support.

5. Encourage Physical Activity and Engagement:

Promote Movement: Encourage gentle exercises or walks to reduce restlessness and improve mood.

Stimulate Cognitive Function: Engage in activities that promote cognitive stimulation, such as puzzles, music, or reminiscence therapy.

6. Monitor and Address Physical Health Needs:

Regular Check-ups: Ensure regular medical assessments to address any underlying health conditions contributing to behavioral changes.

Pain Management: Manage pain effectively to alleviate discomfort and improve overall well-being.

7. Evaluate Medication Management:

Medication Review: Review medications with healthcare providers to assess efficacy and potential side effects.

Adjustments: Adjust dosages or consider alternative treatments to manage behavioral symptoms effectively.

Understanding and managing behavioral changes in individuals with dementia requires a comprehensive approach that addresses underlying causes, environmental influences, and individual needs. By identifying triggers, creating supportive environments, and implementing personalized strategies, caregivers can effectively mitigate behavioral challenges and enhance the quality of life for their loved ones. Collaboration with healthcare professionals, ongoing education, and support from caregiver networks are essential in developing effective management techniques and promoting positive outcomes in dementia care.

Maintaining Relationships

Maintaining relationships while caregiving for someone with dementia is essential for both the caregiver and the person receiving care. This chapter explores strategies and considerations for caregivers to nurture and sustain relationships with their loved ones, family members, friends, and their broader social network despite the challenges posed by dementia.

Understanding Challenges in Relationship Maintenance

1. Communication Difficulties:

Changes in Language: Difficulty finding words, understanding conversations, or expressing thoughts clearly.

Misinterpretations: Challenges in understanding nonverbal cues or responding appropriately.

2. Cognitive Decline:

Memory Loss: Difficulty recalling recent events, names, or familiar faces.

Personality Changes: Shifts in behavior, mood swings, or emotional responses.

3. Role Changes and Dependency:

Shift in Dynamics: Transition from equal partnership to caregiver and care recipient roles.

Increased Dependency: Greater reliance on the caregiver for daily activities and decision-making.

Strategies for Maintaining Relationships

1. Foster Meaningful Interactions:

Spend Quality Time Together: Engage in activities that the person enjoys, such as listening to music, going for walks, or reminiscing about shared experiences.

Create New Traditions: Establish routines or rituals that provide a sense of continuity and connection.

2. Adapt Communication Styles:

Use Simple Language: Speak clearly and calmly, using straightforward sentences to facilitate understanding.

Listen Actively: Practice active listening by paying attention to verbal and nonverbal cues, and responding empathetically.

3. Maintain Social Connections:

Encourage Visits and Communication: Facilitate visits from family members, friends, and social groups to maintain social engagement and support networks.

Use Technology: Utilize video calls, social media, or email to stay connected with distant family members and friends.

4. Educate and Involve Others:

Family and Friends: Educate them about dementia and its impact on relationships, encouraging their involvement and understanding.

Support Groups: Join caregiver support groups or community organizations that provide emotional support and practical advice.

5. Respite and Self-Care:

Take Breaks: Utilize respite care services to allow time for self-care and rejuvenation, preventing caregiver burnout.

Maintain Personal Relationships: Nurture friendships and hobbies outside of caregiving to maintain a sense of identity and fulfillment.

6. Address Challenges and Seek Help:

Professional Support: Consult healthcare professionals, counselors, or dementia specialists for guidance on managing relationship dynamics and addressing behavioral challenges.

Conflict Resolution: Address conflicts or disagreements calmly and constructively, seeking common ground and understanding.

Maintaining relationships while caring for someone with dementia requires patience, adaptability, and proactive efforts to foster meaningful connections. By adapting communication styles, nurturing social connections, and seeking support from others, caregivers can enhance the quality of life for their loved ones and themselves. Building a supportive network, practicing self-care, and educating others about dementia are essential steps in navigating the challenges of caregiving while preserving and strengthening relationships over time. Through compassion, understanding, and effective communication, caregivers can create meaningful moments and maintain meaningful relationships despite the impact of dementia.

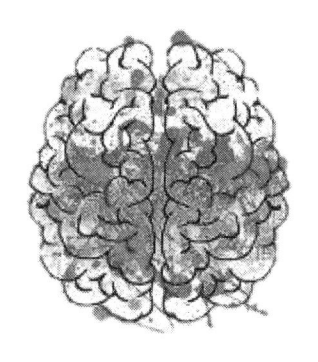

CHAPTER 7:

THERAPHIES AND TREATMENTS

Therapies and treatments for dementia aim to alleviate symptoms, improve quality of life, and support cognitive function for individuals affected by this progressive condition. This chapter explores various therapeutic approaches, medical treatments, and supportive interventions used in the management of dementia.

Pharmacological Treatments

Pharmacological treatments for dementia aim to manage symptoms, slow disease progression, and improve cognitive function and quality of life for individuals affected by various forms of dementia. This chapter explores the medications commonly used in the treatment of dementia, their mechanisms of action, and considerations for their use.

1. Cholinesterase Inhibitors

Cholinesterase inhibitors are the primary class of medications used to treat Alzheimer's disease and some other forms of dementia. They work by increasing the levels of acetylcholine, a neurotransmitter involved in memory and learning, in the brain.

Donepezil (Aricept): Typically prescribed for mild to moderate Alzheimer's disease, it may help improve cognitive symptoms and slow decline in memory and thinking skills.

Rivastigmine (Exelon): Available as a patch or oral formulation, used for mild to moderate Alzheimer's disease and Parkinson's disease dementia.

Galantamine (Razadyne): Used to treat mild to moderate Alzheimer's disease, it also has an effect on nicotinic receptors which may enhance cognition.

Considerations: These medications are generally well-tolerated but may cause side effects such as nausea, vomiting, diarrhea, or insomnia. Regular monitoring is necessary to assess their effectiveness and adjust dosages as needed.

2. Memantine (Namenda)

Memantine is an NMDA receptor antagonist used for moderate to severe Alzheimer's disease. It works by regulating glutamate activity in the brain, which is involved in learning and memory processes.

Mechanism of Action: Memantine helps regulate excess glutamate, which can contribute to neuronal damage in dementia.

Benefits: It may help improve cognitive function, behavior, and daily living activities in individuals with moderate to severe Alzheimer's disease.

Considerations: Memantine is generally well-tolerated, with common side effects including dizziness, headache, confusion, and constipation. It is often used in combination with cholinesterase inhibitors for enhanced therapeutic effect.

3. Antidepressants and Antianxiety Medications

Individuals with dementia may experience mood disturbances such as depression or anxiety, which can impact their overall well-being and quality of life.

Selective Serotonin Reuptake Inhibitors (SSRIs): Examples include sertraline (Zoloft), citalopram (Celexa), and escitalopram (Lexapro), used to manage symptoms of depression and anxiety.

Benzodiazepines: Occasionally prescribed for short-term management of severe anxiety or agitation, but caution is needed due to risks of sedation, confusion, and falls.

Considerations: Careful monitoring is essential when prescribing antidepressants or anxiolytics to individuals with dementia, as they can affect cognition and may interact with other medications.

4. Other Medications

Depending on specific symptoms and individual health needs, healthcare providers may consider other medications or supplements to manage certain aspects of dementia:

Antipsychotic Medications: Used cautiously in cases of severe behavioral symptoms such as aggression, hallucinations, or agitation, but their use is limited due to potential side effects and risks.

Sleep Aids: Prescribed to manage sleep disturbances such as insomnia or disruptions in sleep-wake cycles.

Pain Management: Addressing pain effectively can improve overall comfort and quality of life for individuals with dementia.

5. Individualized Treatment Plans

Treatment for dementia is often individualized based on the type and severity of dementia, as well as the person's overall health, preferences, and response to medications. Regular monitoring by healthcare providers is crucial to assess the effectiveness of treatment, manage side effects, and make adjustments as needed.

Pharmacological treatments play a significant role in managing symptoms and improving quality of life for individuals living with dementia. Cholinesterase inhibitors and memantine are mainstays in the treatment of Alzheimer's disease, targeting cognitive symptoms and disease progression. Antidepressants, anxiolytics, and other medications may be prescribed to address mood disturbances and behavioral symptoms. Careful consideration of individual needs, potential side effects, and regular monitoring are essential aspects of dementia treatment to optimize therapeutic outcomes and enhance overall well-being.

Non-Pharmacological Approaches

Non-pharmacological approaches are essential components of dementia care, focusing on enhancing quality of life, reducing behavioral symptoms, and promoting overall well-being without relying on medications. This chapter explores various non-pharmacological interventions commonly used in the management of dementia.

1. Cognitive Stimulation Therapy (CST)

Cognitive stimulation therapy involves engaging individuals in structured activities and discussions to stimulate cognitive function, memory, and problem-solving skills.

Group Sessions: Facilitated group activities involving puzzles, games, and reminiscence exercises to promote mental stimulation and social interaction.

Benefits: May improve cognitive abilities, communication skills, and mood in individuals with mild to moderate dementia.

2. Reality Orientation Therapy

Reality orientation therapy helps individuals with dementia stay oriented to their surroundings, time, and personal identity through structured interventions.

Orientation Techniques: Using calendars, clocks, and orientation boards to reinforce awareness of time, place, and person.

Benefits: Reduces confusion, enhances feelings of security, and promotes a sense of control and familiarity.

3. Reminiscence Therapy

Reminiscence therapy involves encouraging individuals to discuss past experiences, share stories, and engage in activities that evoke positive memories.

Memory Recall: Using photographs, music, or objects from the past to stimulate reminiscing and emotional connections.

Therapeutic Outcomes: Improves self-esteem, reduces anxiety and depression, and fosters social interaction and communication.

4. Music Therapy

Music therapy utilizes music-based activities to stimulate cognitive function, evoke emotions, and enhance overall well-being in individuals with dementia.

Listening and Singing: Playing familiar music, singing songs, or participating in rhythmic activities to improve mood and reduce agitation.

Benefits: Enhances emotional expression, promotes relaxation, and supports memory recall through music-associated memories.

5. Art Therapy

Art therapy involves engaging individuals in creative activities such as painting, drawing, or sculpting to facilitate self-expression and communication.

Creative Expression: Encourages nonverbal communication and emotional release through artistic mediums.

Therapeutic Benefits: Improves mood, reduces stress and anxiety, and enhances cognitive function through sensory and motor stimulation.

6. Pet Therapy (Animal-Assisted Therapy)

Pet therapy involves interactions with trained animals to provide companionship, comfort, and emotional support to individuals with dementia.

Benefits: Reduces feelings of loneliness and agitation, promotes social interaction, and provides sensory stimulation through tactile and emotional connections with animals.

7. Physical Exercise Programs

Physical exercise programs tailored to the abilities of individuals with dementia can improve physical health, mobility, and overall well-being.

Gentle Exercises: Activities such as walking, stretching, or chair exercises to maintain or improve strength, balance, and flexibility.

Benefits: Enhances cardiovascular health, reduces risk of falls, and promotes better sleep and mood regulation.

8. Environmental Modifications

Creating a supportive and dementia-friendly environment can enhance comfort, safety, and independence for individuals with dementia.

Safety Features: Installing handrails, non-slip flooring, and adequate lighting to prevent accidents and promote mobility.

Sensory Stimulation: Using soothing colors, textures, and familiar objects to create calming or stimulating environments based on individual preferences.

9. Behavioral Management Techniques

Behavioral management strategies help caregivers respond effectively to challenging behaviors such as agitation, aggression, or wandering.

Structured Routine: Establishing predictable daily routines to reduce anxiety and confusion.

Validation and Redirection: Acknowledging emotions, redirecting attention, and using positive reinforcement to manage behavior without resorting to medication.

10. Caregiver Education and Support

Providing education and support to caregivers is crucial for implementing non-pharmacological interventions effectively and improving overall caregiving experiences.

Training Programs: Offering caregivers training in communication techniques, behavioral management strategies, and dementia care principles.

Support Networks: Accessing caregiver support groups, counseling services, or respite care options to reduce stress, share experiences, and enhance coping mechanisms.

Non-pharmacological approaches play a vital role in enhancing the quality of life and managing symptoms for individuals with dementia. By incorporating cognitive stimulation, reality orientation, reminiscence, music, art, and pet therapies, as well as physical exercise and environmental modifications, caregivers can promote well-being and maintain dignity for those affected by dementia. These holistic interventions not only address cognitive and behavioral symptoms but also support emotional, social, and physical health, contributing to a more comprehensive and compassionate approach to dementia care. Regular assessment, individualized planning, and ongoing support from healthcare professionals and caregivers are essential for optimizing the benefits of non-pharmacological interventions throughout the progression of dementia.

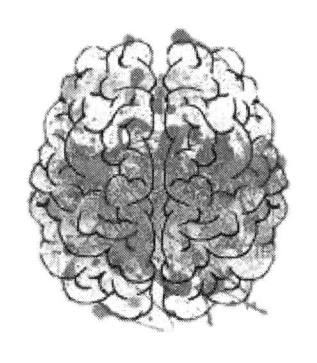

CHAPTER 8:

PREVENTIVE STRATEGIES

Lifestyle Modifications

Lifestyle modifications play a crucial role in managing dementia symptoms, promoting overall brain health, and enhancing quality of life for individuals affected by the condition. This chapter explores key lifestyle changes and interventions that can support cognitive function, emotional well-being, and physical health in individuals with dementia.

1. Physical Exercise

Regular physical activity is beneficial for both brain health and overall well-being in individuals with dementia.

Types of Exercise: Engage in activities such as walking, swimming, gardening, or chair exercises tailored to the individual's abilities.

Benefits: Improves cardiovascular health, enhances circulation to the brain, reduces stress, and promotes better sleep patterns.

2. Healthy Diet

A balanced and nutritious diet can support brain function and overall health in individuals with dementia.

Key Components: Include fruits, vegetables, whole grains, lean proteins (fish, poultry), and healthy fats (olive oil, nuts).

Hydration: Ensure adequate fluid intake to prevent dehydration, which can affect cognition and physical health.

3. Cognitive Stimulation

Engaging in mentally stimulating activities can help maintain cognitive function and stimulate neural pathways.

Activities: Puzzles, crossword puzzles, reading, playing musical instruments, learning new skills or languages.

Social Engagement: Participate in social activities, join clubs, volunteer, or attend community events to promote cognitive stimulation.

4. Sleep Hygiene

Establishing good sleep habits is essential for individuals with dementia to support memory consolidation and overall well-being.

Routine: Maintain a regular sleep schedule, with consistent bedtime and wake-up times.

Environment: Create a comfortable sleep environment with minimal noise and distractions.

5. Stress Management

Reducing stress and managing emotional well-being can improve overall quality of life for individuals with dementia.

Techniques: Practice relaxation techniques such as deep breathing, meditation, yoga, or tai chi.

Support Systems: Seek emotional support from family, friends, support groups, or counseling services.

6. Limiting Alcohol and Avoiding Smoking

Minimizing alcohol consumption and avoiding smoking are important lifestyle choices to protect overall brain and cardiovascular health.

Alcohol: Limit intake to moderate levels as excessive alcohol can impair cognition and interact with medications.

Smoking: Quit smoking to reduce the risk of cardiovascular disease and improve overall health.

7. Safety Measures

Creating a safe environment is crucial to prevent accidents and ensure the well-being of individuals with dementia.

Home Safety: Install grab bars, handrails, non-slip mats, and adequate lighting to reduce fall risks.

Supervision: Ensure constant supervision, especially if wandering or safety concerns arise.

8. Continued Cognitive Assessment and Care Planning

Regular cognitive assessments and care planning are essential to monitor disease progression and adjust interventions accordingly.

Healthcare Team: Collaborate with healthcare professionals to develop personalized care plans based on individual needs and preferences.

Family Involvement: Involve family members in care planning discussions and decision-making processes.

Lifestyle modifications encompass a holistic approach to managing dementia, focusing on promoting brain health, enhancing quality of life, and supporting overall well-being. By incorporating physical exercise, a nutritious diet, cognitive stimulation, stress management techniques, and safety measures, caregivers and individuals with dementia can optimize health outcomes and maintain independence to the greatest extent possible. Ongoing support from healthcare professionals, family members, and community resources plays a crucial role in implementing and sustaining these lifestyle modifications throughout the progression of dementia. Embracing a proactive approach to lifestyle changes can positively impact cognitive function, emotional resilience, and overall quality of life for individuals living with dementia.

Public Health Initiatives

Public health initiatives play a crucial role in raising awareness, promoting prevention strategies, improving care standards, and supporting individuals affected by dementia and their caregivers. This chapter explores key public health initiatives aimed at addressing the growing challenges of dementia on a global scale.

1. Awareness Campaigns

Education and Outreach: Campaigns to educate the public, healthcare professionals, and policymakers about dementia, its symptoms, risk factors, and available resources.

Media and Communication: Utilizing various media platforms to disseminate information, reduce stigma, and encourage early detection and intervention.

2. Early Detection and Diagnosis

Screening Programs: Implementing screening initiatives in healthcare settings to identify early signs of cognitive impairment and dementia.

Training Healthcare Providers: Providing training to healthcare professionals on dementia awareness, diagnosis, and management.

3. Supportive Care and Services

Caregiver Support Programs: Offering education, respite care, counseling, and support groups for caregivers to enhance their skills and well-being.

Community Services: Developing community-based services such as day care centers, memory cafes, and home care support to assist individuals with dementia and their families.

4. Research and Innovation

Funding and Collaboration: Investing in research funding, collaborative networks, and clinical trials to advance understanding of dementia causes, treatments, and potential cures.

Technology and Innovation: Harnessing technological advancements for early detection tools, remote monitoring, and assistive technologies to improve care and quality of life.

5. Policy Development and Advocacy

National Dementia Plans: Developing and implementing national strategies and policies to address dementia care, research, and support services.

Advocacy Efforts: Advocating for increased funding, policy reforms, and legislative support to prioritize dementia as a public health priority.

6. Dementia-Friendly Communities

Community Engagement: Creating dementia-friendly environments through education, training for businesses and public services, and architectural modifications for safety and accessibility.

Inclusion and Empowerment: Promoting social inclusion, participation in community activities, and respecting the rights and dignity of individuals living with dementia.

7. Global Collaboration and Knowledge Sharing

International Cooperation: Collaborating across borders to share best practices, research findings, and resources for a unified global approach to dementia.

Capacity Building: Building capacity in low- and middle-income countries through training, resource allocation, and adaptation of interventions to local contexts.

8. Public Policy and Legal Frameworks

Legal Protections: Establishing legal frameworks to protect the rights and dignity of individuals with dementia, including advance care planning, guardianship, and financial management.

Healthcare Integration: Integrating dementia care into broader healthcare systems to ensure comprehensive and coordinated care across primary, secondary, and tertiary levels.

Public health initiatives for dementia encompass a comprehensive approach to addressing the multifaceted challenges posed by this condition. By raising awareness, enhancing early detection, improving care standards, supporting caregivers, advancing research, and advocating for policy reforms, public health efforts can significantly impact the lives of individuals with dementia and their families worldwide. Continued collaboration, innovation, and commitment from governments, healthcare providers, advocacy organizations, and communities are essential to effectively address the evolving needs of an aging population and ensure dignity, respect, and quality of life for those affected by dementia.

Education and Awareness Campaigns

Education and awareness campaigns are pivotal in increasing understanding, reducing stigma, promoting early detection, and improving support for individuals affected by dementia. This chapter explores the key components and strategies involved in effective education and awareness initiatives.

1. Objectives of Education and Awareness Campaigns

Raise Awareness: Increase public knowledge about dementia, including symptoms, risk factors, and available support services.

Reduce Stigma: Challenge misconceptions and stereotypes associated with dementia to foster a more supportive and inclusive society.

Promote Early Detection: Encourage individuals to recognize early signs of cognitive impairment and seek timely diagnosis and intervention.

Empower Caregivers: Provide caregivers with resources, information, and support to enhance their caregiving skills and well-being.

2. Target Audiences

General Public: Educate community members, families, and individuals about dementia to promote understanding and empathy.

Healthcare Professionals: Provide training and resources to improve dementia awareness, diagnosis, and care practices among healthcare providers.

Policy Makers: Advocate for policies and funding to support dementia research, care services, and public health initiatives.

Schools and Universities: Integrate dementia awareness into educational curricula to raise awareness among future healthcare professionals and the broader community.

3. Key Components of Campaigns

Multimedia Approach: Utilize a variety of platforms and formats, including television, radio, social media, websites, printed materials, and community events.

Personal Stories: Share personal experiences of individuals living with dementia and caregivers to humanize the impact of the disease.

Expert Testimonials: Feature healthcare professionals, researchers, and advocates to provide credible information and advice.

Interactive Workshops and Seminars: Conduct workshops, seminars, and training sessions to educate caregivers, healthcare professionals, and community members.

4. Campaign Strategies

Awareness Weeks or Months: Designate specific periods, such as World Alzheimer's Month (September) or Brain Awareness Week, to focus attention on dementia.

Public Events: Organize community events, health fairs, and awareness walks to engage the public and raise visibility.

Collaborations: Partner with healthcare organizations, advocacy groups, universities, and local businesses to amplify campaign reach and impact.

Targeted Messaging: Tailor messages to different demographics and cultural backgrounds to ensure relevance and effectiveness.

5. Resources and Support

Information Hotlines: Establish hotlines or helplines staffed by trained professionals to provide information, support, and referrals to services.

Online Resources: Develop and maintain comprehensive websites with resources, educational materials, and links to support organizations.

Support Groups: Facilitate support groups for individuals with dementia and their caregivers to share experiences and receive emotional support.

6. Measuring Impact and Evaluation

Surveys and Feedback: Conduct surveys and gather feedback from participants to assess knowledge gained and attitudes changed.

Monitoring Engagement: Track campaign reach, website traffic, social media interactions, and attendance at events to evaluate effectiveness.

Longitudinal Studies: Assess long-term impact on awareness, attitudes, and behaviors related to dementia in the community.

7. Global and Local Initiatives

Global Collaboration: Participate in international campaigns and initiatives to harmonize efforts, share best practices, and advocate for global action on dementia.

Local Adaptation: Customize campaigns to local languages, cultural norms, and healthcare systems to ensure relevance and effectiveness.

Education and awareness campaigns are essential tools in the fight against dementia, empowering individuals, caregivers, healthcare providers, and communities to better understand and respond to the challenges posed by this condition. By raising awareness, reducing stigma, promoting early detection, and fostering supportive environments, these campaigns play a critical role in improving outcomes and quality of life for individuals living with dementia and their families. Continued investment in education, advocacy, and public engagement is vital to sustain momentum, drive policy change, and enhance dementia care and support globally.

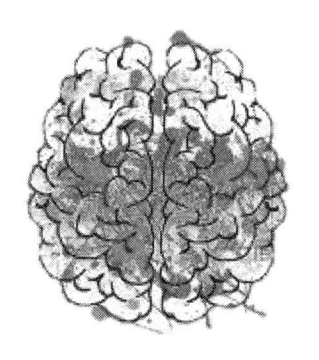

CONCLUSION

Dementia presents a profound and growing challenge for individuals, families, healthcare systems, and societies worldwide. As our understanding of dementia deepens and innovative approaches to care emerge, it is crucial to reflect on the progress made and the path forward in addressing this complex condition.

Progress and Achievements

- Advancements in Research: Significant strides have been made in understanding the underlying causes of dementia, identifying biomarkers, and developing potential treatments aimed at disease modification.
- Enhanced Care Approaches: Person-centered care models, multidisciplinary teams, and technological innovations have transformed dementia care delivery, improving quality of life and support for individuals and caregivers.
- Awareness and Advocacy: Increased public awareness, advocacy efforts, and policy initiatives have reduced stigma, promoted early detection, and prioritized dementia as a global health priority.

Future Directions

- Innovative Therapies: Continued research into disease-modifying treatments, immunotherapies, and neuroprotective agents holds promise for slowing disease progression and improving outcomes.

- Technological Integration: Advancements in telehealth, artificial intelligence, and assistive technologies will further enhance care accessibility, monitoring capabilities, and personalized interventions.
- Global Collaboration: International cooperation, knowledge-sharing, and capacity-building efforts will strengthen healthcare systems and address disparities in dementia care across regions.

Challenges and Opportunities

- Healthcare System Capacity: Addressing workforce shortages, enhancing training for healthcare professionals, and integrating dementia care into primary healthcare settings remain critical challenges.
- Caregiver Support: Providing comprehensive support, education, and respite services for caregivers is essential to alleviate burden and improve caregiver well-being.
- Ethical Considerations: Ensuring ethical standards in research, clinical practice, and decision-making processes related to dementia care, including end-of-life care and legal protections, requires ongoing attention.

The future of dementia care hinges on collaboration, innovation, and a commitment to person-centered approaches that respect individual dignity and autonomy. By leveraging scientific discoveries, embracing technological advancements, and advocating for policy reforms, we can create a more inclusive, supportive environment for individuals living with dementia and their families. Continued investment in research, education, and community engagement is pivotal to realizing our vision of compassionate, effective, and equitable dementia care worldwide.

As we navigate the complexities of dementia, let us strive towards a future where every person affected by this condition receives the respect, support, and quality of life they deserve. Together, we can build a more compassionate and dementia-friendly society where individuals can live with dignity, purpose, and hope.

Made in the USA
Monee, IL
08 July 2024